Posterior Retroperitoneoscopic Adrenalectomy

Carlos Eduardo Costa Almeida
Editor

Posterior Retroperitoneoscopic Adrenalectomy

Indications, Technical Steps
and Outcomes

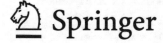 Springer

Editor
Carlos Eduardo Costa Almeida
General Surgery
Portuguese Oncology Institute of Coimbra
Hospital CUF Coimbra
Coimbra, Portugal

ISBN 978-3-031-19997-4   ISBN 978-3-031-19995-0   (eBook)
https://doi.org/10.1007/978-3-031-19995-0

This Springer imprint is published by the registered company Springer Nature Switzerland AG
The registered company address is: Gewerbestrasse 11, 6330 Cham, Switzerland

Preface

Minimally invasive surgery has great advantages for patients compared to open surgery. In adrenal surgery, this is no exception. Although the transperitoneal laparoscopic approach has become the gold standard since its first description in 1992, the posterior retroperitoneoscopic approach provides benefits for both patients and surgeons.

Fifteen years ago, I started using the laparoscopic approach in several different areas, namely colorectal surgery, hepatobiliary surgery, laparoscopic repair of both ventral and groin hernias, and diaphragmatic hernia repair. Since 2005, I have also been using minimally invasive surgery to ligate insufficient lower limbs perforators to heal varicose ulcers. All this has given me a broader perspective of the advantages of every minimally invasive technique.

In 2014, I met Professor Dr. Martin Walz and had my first contact with posterior retroperitoneoscopic adrenalectomy. Not only did I have the opportunity to work with him, but also learned how to perform posterior retroperitoneoscopic adrenalectomy. It was love at first sight, and I immediately thought this great technique could revolutionize adrenal surgery. This approach gives direct access to the adrenal gland, has no incursion into the peritoneal cavity, has minimum risk of viscera injury, and promotes fast recovery. Despite its advantages, many surgeons do not use it because they are not familiar with the retroperitoneum space and are not used to the posterior anatomical perspective. This book will change that.

In 2015, I adopted the posterior retroperitoneoscopic adrenalectomy as the gold standard for adrenal surgery. Since then, I have published data supporting the safety and feasibility of this technique, and I have also proved that a shorter learning curve is possible if surgeons have laparoscopic skills acquired during other procedures. So, there is no reason for surgeons to keep resisting the retroperitoneoscopic approach. In several publications, videos, and scientific lectures, I have tried to demystify the technical difficulties described by some surgeons and contend that learning from an expert is the best way to begin using a new technique.

All the chapters in this book were written by a group of international specialists (surgeons and anesthesiologists) with vast experience in the technique. By sharing their knowledge, they make this book the "expert" a surgeon needs to initiate the "back door" approach to adrenal tumors.

This book intends to provide all general surgeons and urologists interested in adrenal surgery with the knowledge they need to start performing posterior retroperitoneoscopic adrenalectomy safely and effectively. In an easy-to-learn format, it presents the reader with information about anatomical key points, indications for the retroperitoneoscopic approach, possible complications, and limitations of the technique. A step-by-step description with tips and tricks will help surgeons start their adventure in the posterior retroperitoneoscopic approach. The learning curve and the outcomes presented will show the reader why all general surgeons and urologists should prefer this minimally invasive technique. This book aims to contribute to make posterior retroperitoneoscopic adrenalectomy the new gold standard in adrenal surgery.

Coimbra, Portugal   Carlos Eduardo Costa Almeida

Contents

Contributors

Claudia Armellin, MD Endocrine Surgery Unit, Department of Surgery, Oncology and Gastroenterology, University of Padova, Padova, Italy

Stefania Barbieri, MD Department of Medicine, Anesthesiology and Intensive Care, University of Padova, Padova, Italy

Martí Manyalich Blasi, MD General & Digestive Surgery Department, ICMDIM, Hospital Clinic Barcelona, IDIBAPS, University of Barcelona, Barcelona, Spain

Teresa Vieira Caroço, MD General Surgery Department, Portuguese Oncology Institute of Coimbra, Coimbra, Portugal

Michele Carron, MD Department of Medicine, Anesthesiology and Intensive Care, University of Padova, Padova, Italy

Carlos Eduardo Costa Almeida, MD General Surgery, Portuguese Oncology Institute of Coimbra, Hospital CUF Coimbra, Coimbra, Portugal

Varlık Erol, MD Department of General Surgery, Medicana International Hospital, Izmir, Turkey

Paolo Feltracco, MD Department of Medicine, Anesthesiology and Intensive Care, University of Padova, Padova, Italy

Maurizio Iacobone, MD, FEBS/Endocrine Surgery Endocrine Surgery Unit, Department of Surgery, Oncology and Gastroenterology, University of Padova, Padova, Italy

Hugo Louro, MD General Surgery, Centro Hospitalar Vila Nova de Gaia/Espinho, Vila Nova de Gaia, Portugal

Özer Makay, MD, FEBS div Endocrine Surgery Department of General Surgery, Division of Endocrine Surgery, Ege University Hospital, Izmir, Turkey

Murat Özdemir, MD Department of General Surgery, Division of Endocrine Surgery, Ege University Hospital, Izmir, Turkey

David Saavedra-Perez, MD, MSc, FEBS/MIS General & Digestive Surgery Department, ICMDIM, Hospital Clinic Barcelona, IDIBAPS, University of Barcelona, Barcelona, Spain

Carlos Serra, MD, PhD, FACS General Surgery, Hospital dos SAMS, Lisbon, Portugal

Francesca Torresan, MD, PhD Endocrine Surgery Unit, Department of Surgery, Oncology and Gastroenterology, University of Padova, Padova, Italy

Oscar Vidal, MD, PhD, MHM, MPH General & Digestive Surgery Department, ICMDIM, Hospital Clinic Barcelona, IDIBAPS, University of Barcelona, Barcelona, Spain

Jaime Vilaça, MD, PhD, FEBS/MIS General Surgery, Hospital da Luz, Porto, University of Minho, Braga, Porto, Portugal

Abbreviations

ACC	Adrenocortical Carcinoma
ACS	Autonomous Cortisol Hypersecretion
ACTH	Adrenocorticotropic Hormone
AMA	Adrenal Mass Area
APA	Aldosterone Producing Adenoma
ARR	Aldosterone/Renin Ratio
ASA	American Society of Anesthesiologists
AVS	Adrenal Venous Sampling
BMI	Body Mass Index
COPD	Chronic Obstructive Pulmonary Disease
CT	Computed Tomography
DFI	Disease-Free Interval
DFS	Disease-Free Survival
DHEAS	Dehydroepiandrosterone Sulfate
DOTA	Dodecane Tetraacetic Acid
EBL	Estimated Blood Loss
ENSAT	European Network for the Study of Adrenal Tumors
ESES	European Society of Endocrine Surgeons
ETCO$_2$	End-Tidal CO$_2$
FDA	Fluorodopamine
FDG	Fluorodeoxyglucose
FDOPA	Fluorodihydroxyphenylalanine
HLOS	Hospital Length of Stay
HU	Hounsfield Unit
ICU	Intensive Care Unit
IVC	Inferior Vena Cava
LA	Laparoscopic Approach
LAdr	Laparoscopic Adrenalectomy
LFS	Li-Fraumeni Syndrome
LPRA	Laparoscopic Posterior Retroperitoneal Adrenalectomy
MEN	Multiple Endocrine Neoplasia
METs	Metabolic Equivalents
MIAS	Minimally Invasive Adrenal Surgery
MRI	Magnetic Resonance Imaging
NF-1	Neurofibromatosis Type-1
NSCLC	Non-Small Cell Lung Cancer
OA	Open Approach

PA	Primary Aldosteronism
PBMH	Primary Bilateral Macronodular Hyperplasia
PET	Positron-Emission Tomography
PFT	Pulmonary Function Testing
PONV	Postoperative Nausea and Vomiting
PPGL	Pheochromocytoma and Paraganglioma
PPNAD	Primary Pigmented Nodular Adrenocortical Disease
PRA	Posterior Retroperitoneoscopic Adrenalectomy
RA	Retroperitoneoscopic Approach
RFA	Retroperitoneal Fat Area
RPRA	Robotic Posterior Retroperitoneal Adrenalectomy
TL-RA	Transabdominal Lateral Robotic Adrenalectomy
TLA	Transperitoneal Laparoscopic Approach
TLAdr	Transperitoneal Laparoscopic Adrenalectomy
VAS	Visual Analog Scale
VHL	von Hippel-Lindau

Anatomy of the Adrenal Gland

Teresa Vieira Caroço
and Carlos Eduardo Costa Almeida

1.1 Introduction

The adrenal glands are paired organs located above the kidneys. Their name derives from the Latin expression *ad renalis*, meaning "of the kidneys" [1, 2]. They are also occasionally referred to as "suprarenal glands" [3]. The first description of the adrenal is attributed to Galeno, but it was only in the sixteenth century that Bartolomeus Eustachius provided its first complete description and illustration [2].

Adrenals are complex endocrine structures, secreting hormones that are essential to maintaining body function. They produce two types of hormones, each one originating from a different layer. The outer layer of the adrenal, called *cortex*, secretes steroid hormones of three major categories: [1, 3].

1. Mineralocorticoids (aldosterone), regulate salt and volume homeostasis.
2. Glucocorticoids (cortisol), regulate glucose usage, as well as both immune and inflammatory homeostasis.
3. Androgens (dehydroepiandrosterone sulfate (DHEAS)), play an important role in fetoplacental estrogen synthesis. They also serve as substrate for peripheral androgen synthesis in women.

The inner layer, called *medulla*, is part of the sympathetic nervous system. It secretes catecholamines (epinephrine and norepinephrine), acting as rapid responses to stress to regulate multiple physiological parameters, such as cardiac output [1, 3]. The physiological processes through which all the hormones are produced fall beyond the scope of this chapter.

The two distinguished layers of the adrenal gland have different embryological origins. The cortex is derived from the mesodermal cells in the vicinity of the formatting kidney, starting in the fourth week of gestation, whereas medulla derives from the ectodermal neural crest cells [1, 2, 4]. The cells from the ectodermal neural crest, also known as *chromaffin cells* due to their staining properties, migrate to the cortex in the seventh week of gestation, and gradually invade it until achieving their definitive location in the center of the gland, the medulla. This migration of cells explains the existence of heterotopic adrenal glands and paragangliomas, mainly para-aortic and paravertebral [4].

T. V. Caroço (✉)
General Surgery Department, Portuguese Oncology Institute of Coimbra, Coimbra, Portugal

C. E. Costa Almeida
General Surgery, Portuguese Oncology Institute of Coimbra, Hospital CUF Coimbra, Coimbra, Portugal
e-mail: carloscostaalmeida@yahoo.com

© The Author(s), under exclusive license to Springer Nature Switzerland AG 2023
C. E. Costa Almeida (ed.), *Posterior Retroperitoneoscopic Adrenalectomy*,
https://doi.org/10.1007/978-3-031-19995-0_1

1.2   The Adrenal Gland

The adrenal glands are two retroperitoneal organs, one on the right and one on the left side, located in the superomedial portion of the kidney [4–7]. The adrenals have a yellow-grayish color and firm consistency. Although they may vary in volume, they usually weigh 4–8 g, measure 4–5 cm in length and 2–4 cm in width. The right adrenal has a pyramidal/triangular shape, it is in a higher position over the kidney, and behind the inferior vena cava (IVC) [8]. The left adrenal is more semilunar shaped and lies superiorly and anteromedially to the kidney. Both glands are surrounded by the perirenal fat and enclosed in the perirenal fascia, except for the area of connective tissue that separates them from the kidney. Fibrous bands attach the glands to the abdominal wall and diaphragm [4–6] (Fig. 1.1).

1.2.1   Anatomical Landmarks and Topographic Anatomy

The adrenal glands are located laterally to each side of the spine, encased by the 10th, 11th, and 12th ribs on the left, and the 11th and 12th ribs on the right. The right adrenal is in a lower position than the left gland [4, 8]. Both glands are in close relation with the diaphragmatic crura. Their anatomical relations are different on each side, which implies important considerations in the surgical approach (Fig. 1.1). In both glands, we can consider an anterior and a posterior surface [4, 5, 7, 8].

- Right adrenal gland—The anterior surface of the right adrenal contacts with the IVC, separated only by a thin layer of fascia and connective tissue. The IVC is in front and medial to the adrenal, but it sometimes covers the gland

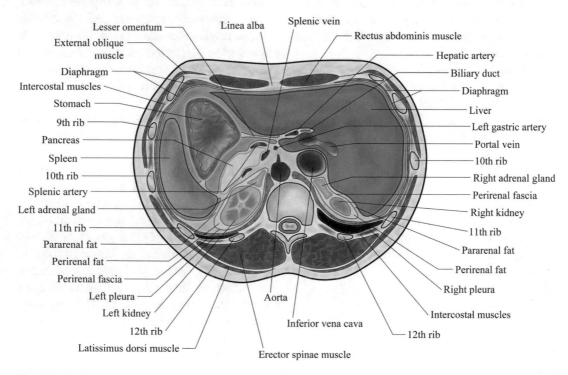

Fig. 1.1 Axial plane showing the anatomical relations of both the adrenals

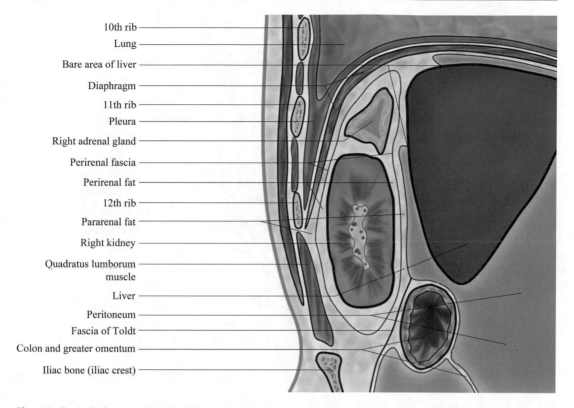

10th rib
Lung
Bare area of liver
Diaphragm
11th rib
Pleura
Right adrenal gland
Perirenal fascia
Perirenal fat
12th rib
Pararenal fat
Right kidney
Quadratus lumborum muscle
Liver
Peritoneum
Fascia of Toldt
Colon and greater omentum
Iliac bone (iliac crest)

Fig. 1.2 Sagittal plane crossing the right adrenal gland

entirely [4, 5]. This major vein separates the anterior surface of the gland from the Winslow foramen, the second part of the duodenum, and the head of the pancreas. The lateral upper part of the anterior surface of the gland is in close relation with the bare area of the liver, while the inferolateral part is covered by the peritoneum, the liver, and hepatic flexure of the colon [8]. The posterior surface is divided by a ridge. The superior border rests in contact with the diaphragm, and the inferior surface is in contact with the right kidney [4, 5]. The right adrenal is not close to the renal vessels due to its high suprarenal position (Fig. 1.2).

- Left adrenal gland—Superiorly, the anterior surface is in close relation with the peritoneum of the posterior wall of the lesser sac (omental bursa), which separates the gland from the spleen and stomach. Inferiorly, the anterior surface is not covered by peritoneum but by the body/tail of the pancreas and splenic vessels (artery and vein). As for the right adre-

nal, the posterior surface of the left adrenal contacts with the diaphragmatic crus [8]. Medially, the left adrenal gland is about 7 mm away from the aorta. Contrasting with the right adrenal, the left adrenal lies partially in front of the kidney and because of that, it is close to the left renal vein [8] (Fig. 1.3).

In the most medial/inner area of both adrenals are the splanchnic nerves major and minor and the semilunar ganglia, as well as the inferior phrenic artery, bilaterally. In this inner area, the adrenals are closely united to the prerenal fascia and therefore, it is very difficult to lift the gland without opening this fascia [4, 5].

1.2.2   Arterial Supply

The adrenals are highly vascularized organs with one of the highest flow rates, up to 10 ml/min. Their vascularization is unique [2, 4, 5]. The arte-

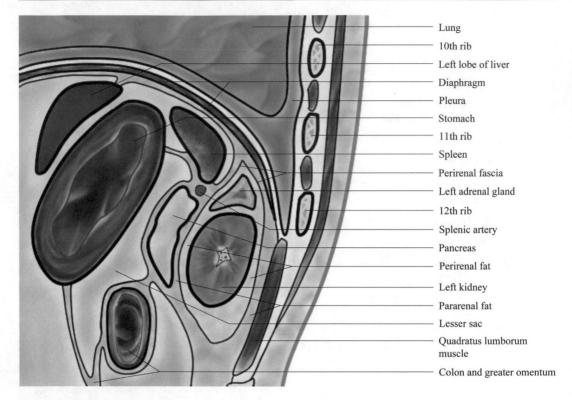

Lung
10th rib
Left lobe of liver
Diaphragm
Pleura
Stomach
11th rib
Spleen
Perirenal fascia
Left adrenal gland
12th rib
Splenic artery
Pancreas
Perirenal fat
Left kidney
Pararenal fat
Lesser sac
Quadratus lumborum muscle
Colon and greater omentum

Fig. 1.3 Sagittal plane crossing the left adrenal gland

rial supply derives from three main sources, being identical on both sides [7, 8] (Fig. 1.4).

1. Superior adrenal arteries: several arteries (usually one to three) originating from the inferior phrenic artery, before supplying the diaphragm.
2. Medial adrenal artery: originating directly from the aorta, above the origin of the renal artery. It reaches the inner side of the adrenal and branches both surfaces of the gland. On the right side, those rami cross the IVC in a retrocaval position. This artery is inconstant.
3. Inferior adrenal artery: originating from the renal artery, it enters the gland in its inferior surface.

Besides these three main sources, the adrenal glands may also be supplied by small arteries originating from the subcostal and gonadal vessels. There can be up to 50 arterioles, forming a complex plexus under the adrenal capsule [8].

1.2.3 Venous Drainage

The venous system has no analogy with the arterial system, and it is not consistent on both sides. Most of the times, each gland has one single adrenal vein. Whereas on the right, the major adrenal vein is short (5 mm) and collects blood from the gland and drains directly into the IVC, the left adrenal vein is longer (30 mm), emerges in the adrenal hilum, and runs inferomedially to join the inferior phrenic vein, before draining into the left renal vein [7, 8] (Fig. 1.4). Other small accessory veins may be found in about 5–10% of patients: on the right side, they may drain into the IVC, the right hepatic vein, or the right renal vein, and on the left side, they may drain into the inferior phrenic vein, or the left renal vein [8].

Anatomical variations of the right adrenal vein have been described in 12.8% of patients [9]; on the contrary, anatomical variations are rare on the left side. As described above, the

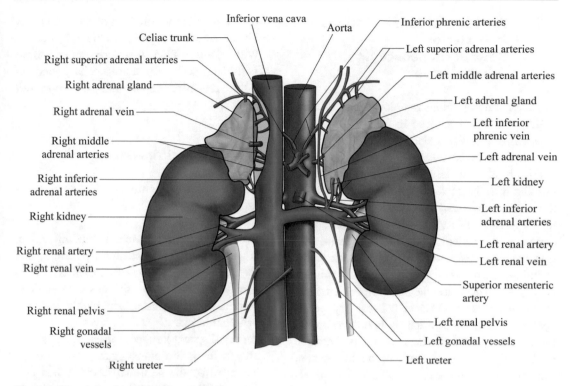

Fig. 1.4 Vascularization of the adrenal glands

right adrenal vein usually drains into the IVC in about 87.6% of patients. Possible anatomical variations are an adrenal vein draining into a posterior hepatic vein in 1.6% of cases, an adrenal vein draining into the IVC just caudal to a hepatic vein in 6.3%, two adrenal veins draining into the IVC in 3.1% of patients, or one adrenal vein draining into the IVC immediately cranial to the renal vein [9].

1.2.4   Lymphatic Drainage

One lymphatic plexus is found inside the adrenal capsule, and a second lymphatic plexus is in the medulla [8]. Both lymphatic plexuses drain to the renal hilar lymph nodes, paraaortic lymph nodes near the diaphragmatic crura and renal artery, and paracaval lymph nodes. Additionally, some lymphatic vessels can cross the diaphragm through small orifices that contain the splanchnic nerves, and drain into the ductus thoracicus, prevertebral

lymph nodes, and posterior mediastinal lymph nodes [2–5]. This lymphatic drainage justifies the location of distant metastases in cases of adrenal cancer [8].

1.2.5   Innervation

The innervation of the adrenals originates in the celiac plexus, the renal plexus, and the thoracic splanchnic nerves [4, 5]. The adrenal plexus can be grouped in three secondary plexuses, depending on the origin of the nerve fibers: adrenoceliac plexus; adrenorenal plexus; adrenodiaphragmatic plexus [5]. Because the adrenal plexus is found between the inner aspect of each gland and the celiac and aortorenal ganglia, they are mainly preganglionic sympathetic fibers that synapse in the medullary chromaffin cells. Although in smaller proportion, postganglionic sympathetic nerve fibers do exist, to innervate the cortical blood vessels [4, 5].

1.3 Anatomical Considerations in Posterior Retroperitoneoscopic Adrenalectomy

Posterior retroperitoneoscopic adrenalectomy (PRA) was first described in 1994 [10–12] and standardized by Prof. Martin Walz in 2001 [13]. PRA has several advantages over the laparoscopic approach. Nevertheless, surgeons are usually not familiar with the posterior anatomical perspective, the reason why many still prefer the transperitoneal approach. For PRA, which is a "backdoor" approach, the patient is positioned in prone position and the incisions are made in the back. In this technique, there is no incursion into the peritoneal cavity, which decreases the risk of injuries to intra-abdominal viscera. Whether using a transperitoneal or a retroperitoneal approach, the anatomy of the adrenals and their surroundings is the same, but the surgeon must be aware of the different and smaller working space in the latter. In their minds, surgeons must shift from the anterior anatomical perspective towards a posterior anatomical view. When entering the retroperitoneum through the "backdoor" approach, surgeons directly access the perirenal fascia, the perirenal fat, and the posterior surfaces of both the kidney and the adrenal gland (Fig. 1.1).

In a posterior view, the right adrenal gland covers the posterior surface of the IVC. From this posterior anatomical perspective, the right adrenal vein stands behind the adrenal, between the gland and the IVC. Dissection and mobilization of the right adrenal is necessary to conduct a careful identification and ligation of the right adrenal vein. On the left side, the left adrenal vein will be identified in the inferomedial border of the gland. Due to its anatomical position, dissection and ligation of the left adrenal vein is much easier than that of the right adrenal vein (Fig. 1.4).

To dissect the adrenals from the upper pole of the kidneys, it is necessary to push the kidneys down. The left adrenal falls in front of the upper part of the anterior surface of the kidney, which means that from a posterior perspective, the left kidney will be in front of the lower pole of the adrenal. In conclusion, to dissect the entire left adrenal, a greater mobilization of the left kidney will be necessary, comparing to the right side.

With regard to PRA, there are some anatomical considerations to be made especially concerning the retroperitoneum and the posterior abdominal wall.

1.3.1 Retroperitoneum

The retroperitoneum is divided into three compartments [4]:

- Anterior pararenal space: ascending colon, descending colon, duodenum, pancreas, and root of the small bowel mesentery. It is bounded anteriorly by the posterior parietal peritoneum and posteriorly by the anterior perirenal fascia.
- Perirenal space: kidneys, adrenal glands, and ureters in their upmost part. This space is delimited by the perirenal fascia. When performing PRA, the surgeon will be working in this area, after passing the posterior pararenal space.
- Posterior pararenal space: bounded anteriorly by the posterior perirenal fascia and posteriorly by the posterior abdominal wall muscles, namely quadratus lumborum, transversus abdominis, and the thoracolumbar fascia. This space contains no organs and is the first area surgeons enter during PRA on their way to the perirenal space.

These retroperitoneal spaces are separated by avascular interfascial planes. These spaces and planes extend through the posterior midline, are adjacent to the bare area of the liver and hemidiaphragms, and fuse together in the pelvis. Due to these features, there is a route for thoracic and pelvis dissemination (e.g., fluids) [4].

During PRA, the surgeon goes through the abdominal wall lateral to the lumboiliac area, passes the posterior pararenal space, and directly enters the perirenal space. Since there are no organs in the posterior pararenal space, there is minimal risk of inadvertent injury to viscera when preforming the "backdoor" approach.

1.3.2 Abdominal Wall (Posterior and Anterolateral)

The abdomen has a superior wall (the diaphragm), a posterior wall, and an anterolateral wall [14]. The aim of this chapter is to provide a brief description of the muscles compounding the lumboiliac area and anterolateral wall. An exhaustive anatomical description falls beyond the scope of this chapter.

The posterior abdominal wall includes the spine and two lumboiliac areas. The lumboiliac area is limited superiorly by the 12th rib, laterally by the lateral border of the quadratus lumborum, inferiorly by the iliac crest, and medially by the spine. This area has three groups of muscles and is the medial landmark for performing PRA. From a posterior anatomical perspective, we will describe the groups from posterior to anterior. The posterior group contains the latissimus dorsi muscle and its aponeurosis, the serratus posterior inferior muscle, and the erector spinae muscle. The middle group is formed by the posterior insertion of the transversus muscle aponeurosis and by the intertransverse processes muscles. The anterior group lies in front of the transversus aponeurosis and contains the quadratus lumborum and the psoas muscles [15]. The thoracolumbar fascia is a thin fibrous layer covering all these muscles, and it is divided in three layers. The anterior layer covers the quadratus lumborum; the medium and posterior layers encase the erector spinae muscle and fuse in a strong raphe at the lateral border of this muscle. This raphe is joined by the anterior layer to form the aponeurosis of the transversus abdominis muscle at the lateral border of the quadratus lumborum [4]. During PRA, the lumboiliac area (specially the erector spinae muscle) is the medial landmark for trocar positioning.

The anterolateral wall of the abdomen is formed by the rectus abdominis, the pyramidal, the transversus abdominis, the internal oblique, and the external oblique muscles. While performing PRA, surgeons work only in the posterior half of the anterolateral wall of the abdomen. This area has three large muscles (outer to inner): external oblique muscle, internal oblique muscle, and transversus abdominis muscle, all separated by thin layers of cellular tissue. The fascia transversalis covers the deep surface of the transversus abdominis muscle almost entirely. In the front, these muscles end in aponeurotic membranes that encase the rectus abdominis muscles and form the linea alba in the middle [7, 14].

The superior lumbar triangle, or triangle of Grynfelt (Fig. 1.5), is usually pierced by the medial trocar during PRA. This triangle is bounded laterally by the posterior border of the internal oblique muscle, medially by the lateral border of the spine muscles, and superiorly by the 12th rib. Sometimes, the triangle becomes square-shaped if the serratus posterior inferior muscle covers the angle between the 12th rib and the spine muscles. In this triangle, the transversus abdominis aponeurosis is directly covered by the latissimus dorsi muscle [7, 15]. The triangle of Grynfeltt is a point of weakness of the abdominal wall and an area of herniation. Because the medial half of the triangle is covered anteriorly by the quadratus lumborum, the true weak point is the lateral half, where the transversus abdominis aponeurosis is perforated by vessels and nerves [15].

The inferior lumbar triangle, or triangle of Petit (Fig. 1.5), is another area of weakness and herniation that can be found when the latissimus dorsi muscle does not extend to the external oblique muscle. The boundaries of this triangle are the posterior border of the external oblique muscle, laterally, the latissimus dorsi, medially, and the iliac bone, inferiorly [7, 15]. The triangle of Petit is not usually punctured during PRA.

The blood supply of the posterior abdominal wall derives from dorsal branches of the intercostal arteries, lumbar arteries, and lateral sacral arteries [4]. Important vessels of the anterolateral wall are the superior and inferior epigastric vessels, and the deep circumflex iliac vessels. There are also some non-significant ramifications of intercostal and lumbar vessels [14]. When performing PRA, there is no risk of causing injury to any of these vascular structures.

The skin of the back is innervated by the posterior rami of the spinal nerves. Midline posterior incisions may cause temporary peri-incisional

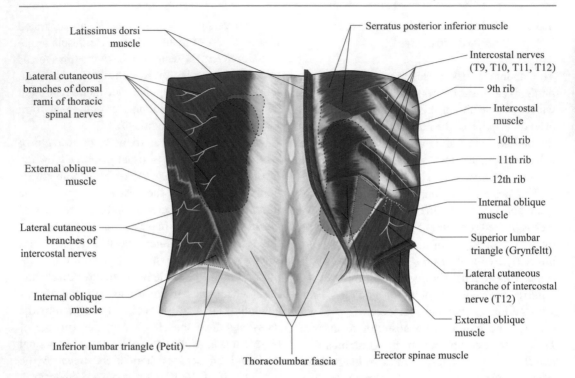

Fig. 1.5 Posterior view of the abdominal wall muscles and nerves. The projection of the adrenals protected by the lower ribs is shown

numbness, which will disappear over time like elsewhere in the body [4]. The intercostal nerves are the ventral (or anterior) rami of the spinal nerves. They run along the inferior border of the ribs, below the intercostal artery, originating muscular branches for the intercostal muscles, and cutaneous branches (lateral and anterior). In front of the mid-axillar line, the lateral cutaneous branch perforates the intercostal muscles and emerges from the abdominal wall muscles to innervate the teguments [16]. The intercostal T12 nerve is subcostal, not intercostal. It runs along the inferior border of the 12th rib, initially in front of the quadratus lumborum, and then it goes between the transversus abdominis and the internal oblique muscle [14, 16]; afterwards, it follows the same distribution of other intercostal nerves. The lateral cutaneous branch of the intercostal T12 nerve arises near the border of the quadratus lumborum, perforates the abdominal wall muscles, and becomes subcutaneous at the level of the middle part of the iliac crest; it originates several branches responsible for sensory innervation of the teguments over the hip and the

gluteal region [16]. Care must be taken with horizontal incisions and large bites of suture which can encase or transect the nerves supplying motor innervation, rising the risk for hernias or pseudo-hernias [4].

Figure 1.5 illustrates the posterior abdominal wall, the posterior half of the anterolateral wall, and the relative position of the kidneys and adrenals in front of the muscles. The adrenals are protected by the 10th, 11th, and 12th ribs. When entering the retroperitoneum below the 12th rib, care must be taken to avoid injury to the intercostal nerve T12 and the consequent abdominal wall relaxation and/or hypoesthesia. The anatomical position of the gland is what dictates how we place the trocars in the "backdoor" approach (see Chap. 7). In PRA, the muscles of the abdominal wall that are crossed through are the latissimus dorsi, the external oblique, the internal oblique, and the transversus abdominis. The paravertebral muscles as the erector spinae and quadratus lumborum are usually not injured during the procedure, as they are the limit for the medial trocar placement.

References

1. Koeppen BM, Stanton BA. The adrenal gland. In: Koeppen BM, Stanton BA, editors. Berne and levy physiology. 7th ed. Philadelphia, PA: Elsevier; 2018. p. 766–86.
2. Visser B, Krampitz GW. The spleen and adrenal glands. In: Parks RW, editor. Hepatobiliary and pancreatic surgery: a companion to specialist surgical practice. 6th ed. USA: Elsevier; 2019. p. 168–79.
3. Holt EH, Lupsa B, Lee GS, Bassyouni H, Peery HE. The adrenal glands. In: Holt EH, Lupsa B, Lee GS, Bassyouni H, Peery HE, editors. Goodman's basic medical endocrinology. 5th ed. Elsevier; 2022. p. 101–43.
4. Degirolamo K, Melck AL. Adrenal glands. In: Brennan PA, Standring MS, Wiseman SM, editors. Gray's surgical anatomy. 1st ed. Elsevier; 2020. p. 486–90.
5. Rouvière H, Delmas A. Organos lumbares: cápsulas o glándulas suprarrenales. In: Rouvière H, Delmas A, editors. Anatomía Humana: descriptiva, topográfica y funcional. 9th ed. Masson; 1996. p. 519–24.
6. Munver R, Stites J. Surgical and radiographic anatomy of the adrenals. In: Partin AW, Dmochowski RR, Kavoussi LR, Peters C, editors. Campbell-Walsh-Wein urology. 12th ed. Philadelphia, PA: Elsevier; 2021. p. 2345–53.
7. Netter F. Atlas of human anatomy. 2nd ed. New Jersey: Novartis; 1997.
8. Uludag M, Aygün N, Isgör A. Surgical indications and techniques for adrenalectomy. SiSli Etfal Hastan Tip Bul. 2020;54(1):8–22.
9. Walz M. Posterior retroperitoneoscopic adrenalectomy. In: Dimitros L, van Heerden JA, editors. Adrenal glands diagnostic aspects and surgical therapy. Berlin, Heidelberg: Springer; 2005. p. 333–9.
10. Johansson K, Anderberg B, Asberg B. Endoscopic retroperitoneal adrenalectomy. A technique useful for surgery of minor tumors. Lakartidningen. 1994;91(37):3278–81.
11. Whittle DE, Schroeder D, Purchas SH, Sivakumaran P, Conaglen JV. Laparoscopic retroperitoneal left adrenalectomy in a patient with Cushin's syndrome. Aust N Z J Surg. 1994;64(5):375–6.
12. Uchida M, Imaide Y, Yoneda K, Uehara H, Ukimura O, Itoh Y, et al. Endoscopic adrenalectomy by retroperitoneal approach for primary aldosteronism. Hinyokika Kiyo. 1994;40(1):43–6.
13. Walz MK, Peitgen K, Walz MV, Hoermann R, Saller B, Giebler RM, et al. Posterior retroperitoneoscopic adrenalectomy: lessons learned within five years. World J Surg. 2001;25(6):728–34.
14. Rouvière H, Delmas A. Anatomía Topográfica del Abdomen. In: Rouvière H, Delmas A, editors. Anatomía Humana: descriptiva, topográfica y funcional. 9th ed. Masson; 1996. p. 481–504.
15. Rouvière H, Delmas A, Región Lumbar Y. Pelvis menor. In: Rouvière H, Delmas A, editors. Anatomía Humana: descriptiva, topográfica y funcional. 9th ed. MASSON; 1996. p. 505–18.
16. Rouvière H, Delmas A. Nervios del tronco. In: Rouvière H, Delmas A, editors. Anatomía Humana: descriptiva, topográfica y funcional. 9th ed. Masson; 1996. p. 254–79.

Indications for Adrenalectomy

Carlos Serra

2.1 Introduction

The history of adrenal surgery dates back to 1914, when Perry Sargent performed the first planned adrenalectomy, followed by Charles Mayo in 1927 with the first flank approach to pheochromocytoma [1].

Laparoscopic adrenalectomy, described for the first time by Gagner, in 1992, rapidly became the gold standard for treating benign adrenal pathology [2]. As experience in this surgery increased, even some malignant diseases are amenable to laparoscopic resection without compromising the oncological outcome and having the benefits of the minimally invasive procedure [1].

In its current approach by Martin Walz, posterior retroperitoneoscopic adrenalectomy (PRA) was worldwide popularized as an effective alternative to laparoscopic adrenalectomy. This technique adds the advantages of the prior posterior approach with those of minimally invasive surgery, namely a more direct approach to the retroperitoneum and a simple access to the adrenal gland without the need to mobilize intra-abdominal organs [3]. Differently from transperitoneal laparoscopic adrenalectomy (TLAdr), where the working space is immediately obtained with gas insufflation, in PRA, the working space must be created [4]. All indications for laparoscopic adrenalectomy are nowadays also indications for the posterior retroperitoneoscopic approach [5]. Posterior approach has obvious advantages in patients with multiple prior abdominal surgeries since it provides an adhesion-free surgical field.

In general terms, there are two indications for the surgical removal of the adrenal glands: malignancy (or suspicion of malignancy) and hormonal overproduction caused by an adrenal tumor. Even though malignant adrenal tumors, especially adrenocortical tumors, are usually treated with open surgery, malignancy is not an absolute contraindication for minimally invasive surgery.

In this chapter, we describe the indications for adrenalectomy, emphasizing the advantages and disadvantages of PRA in contrast with the more common TLAdr.

2.2 Posterior Retroperitoneoscopic Adrenalectomy in Overproduction Adrenal Syndromes

Overproduction adrenal syndromes can affect any of the hormones produced by the adrenal glands: aldosterone, cortisol, catecholamines, or

C. Serra (✉)
General Surgery, Hospital dos SAMS,
Lisbon, Portugal
e-mail: carlos.serra@sams.pt

sexual hormones. Overproduction of sexual hormones is usually associated with malignancy so it will be described in that section.

2.2.1 Excessive Production of Aldosterone: Hyperaldosteronism

Aldosterone, the major mineralocorticoid steroid hormone, is secreted from zona glomerulosa of the adrenal cortex, and its primary effect is the uptake and retention of sodium and water, with potassium and hydrogen excretion acting in the distal convoluted tubules of kidney, gastrointestinal mucosa, salivary and sweat glands [6]. Hyperaldosteronism may be classified as primary or secondary, depending on the underlying causes (Table 2.1).

Primary aldosteronism (PA)—Conn's syndrome—represents the autonomous secretion of aldosterone from either one or both adrenal glands, independent of its primary regulators: angiotensin II, hyperkalemia, and adrenocorticotropic hormone (ACTH) [7]. The first description of the disease was written by Jerome W. Conn in 1955 [8].

PA is the most common cause of endocrine hypertension, with a prevalence of 6% in the general hypertensive population and 12% in severe cases of hypertension. It carries an increased risk of adverse health outcomes, which justifies screening of risky patients (Table 2.2), and an aggressive normalization of aldosterone [7]. Classic manifestations of PA include hypertension, hypokalemia, and metabolic alkalosis [9].

The most recommended screening test for PA is the Aldosterone/Renin Ratio (ARR) measured under standard conditions, with a value >30 ng/dl considered positive (with serum aldosterone level > 15 ng/dl) [7]. A positive screening test must be confirmed by one of the four confirmatory tests: oral sodium loading, saline infusion, fludrocortisone suppression, or captopril challenge [7].

PA may be caused by unilateral involvement, an aldosterone-producing adenoma (APA), which is considered a surgically curable disease, or

Table 2.1 Causes of hyperaldosteronism

Causes of primary hyperaldosteronism	
Aldosterone-producing adenoma	35%
Bilateral idiopathic adrenal hyperplasia	60%
Primary unilateral adrenal hyperplasia	2%
Pure aldosterone-producing adrenocortical carcinoma	<1%
Familiar aldosteronism	<1%
Type 1—Glucocorticoid remediable	<2%
Type 2—Familiar aldosteronism or hyperplasia	
Ectopic aldosterone-producing adenoma/carcinoma	<0.1%
Causes of secondary hyperaldosteronism	
Edema disorders 1. Cardiac failure 2. Liver failure / cirrhosis 3. Nephrotic syndrome	
States of reduced renal perfusion 1. Renal artery stenosis 2. Advanced atherosclerosis 3. Malignant hypertension	
Renin-producing tumors	
Pregnancy	

Table 2.2 Indications for screening for primary hyperaldosteronism

Early onset of hypertension (< 20 years)
Hypertension resistant to two or more antihypertensive drugs
Severe hypertension (systolic bp > 160 or diastolic bp > 100 mmHg)
Hypertension with spontaneous hypokalemia (or secondary to low-dose diuretic)
Adrenal incidentaloma
Evaluation for secondary causes of hypertension
Familiar history of hypertension and primary hyperaldosteronism

bilateral involvement (idiopathic adrenal hyperplasia), considered non-amenable to surgical cure. Recent studies have reported new variants of surgically treatable PA, including diffuse or nodular unilateral hyperplasia [10].

Distinguishing between bilateral or unilateral hypersecretion is crucial since only the latter is amenable to surgical cure. For this purpose, several techniques can be used: adrenal venous sampling (AVS), magnetic resonance imaging (MRI), computed tomography (CT), and adrenocortical scintigraphy [7]. AVS is an invasive procedure, with a low risk of complications (0.6%) for skilled radiologists, and a failure rate between 3 and 22%, yet superior to image-based techniques for surgical decision, namely identifying non-nodular unilateral hyperplasia [11].

Surgery is the treatment of choice in APA or other unilateral PA variants, since it provides the best blood pressure control, with an increase in patients' quality of life [7]. Minimally invasive surgery, either by transperitoneal (laparoscopic) or retroperitoneal approach, is, nowadays, the most popular strategy to treat patients with unilateral PA [7].

Hypokalemia is resolved in nearly all patients with APA after unilateral adrenalectomy. Hypertension is cured (no need for medication) in 30–35% of APA patients after unilateral adrenalectomy or subtotal resections, although hypertension improves in about 90% of them [12]. Some preoperative factors increase the likelihood of resolution of hypertension: fewer than three antihypertensive medications, younger age, female gender, shorter duration of hypertension, and lower body mass index (BMI) [12].

According to two meta-analyses comparing transperitoneal and retroperitoneal adrenalectomy, both techniques have similar outcomes, though a third meta-analysis claimed better short-term outcomes for the retroperitoneal approach (RA) [13]. Characteristics of patients and adenomas associated with Conn's syndrome make this disease particularly amenable to RA:

- patients are usually thin, without the amount of retroperitoneal fat associated with other adrenal diseases, which facilitates dissection.
- Conn's adenomas are generally small lesions, with dimensions that do not create the lack of space problems associated with bigger tumors.

As the most dissuasive arguments used against PRA are the absence of obvious anatomical landmarks in the retroperitoneal space, caused by the great amount of fat and the short working field, patients with PA are ideal for the PRA-initiating surgeon after proper training and mentoring. Some patients with APA are amenable to partial adrenalectomy, without compromising the outcome. Indications for partial adrenalectomy will be discussed in another section of this chapter.

2.2.2 Excessive Production of Glucocorticoids: Cushing's Syndrome

Since its first description by Harvey Cushing, in 1932, Cushing's syndrome or hypercortisolism has been a complex disease presenting diagnostic and therapeutic dilemmas [14]. Cushing's syndrome (endogenous hypercortisolism) is characterized by increased levels of circulating glucocorticoids and can be divided into two types [15]:

- ACTH dependent, caused by pituitary or ectopic ACTH secretion, representing the majority of patients
- ACTH independent, due to an autonomous adrenal excessive production of corticosteroids from zona fasciculata, which accounts for 20–30% of patients with endogenous hypercortisolism (10–15% adenomas, 5–10% carcinomas, 5% hyperplasia) [15]

Endogenous hypercortisolism is a rare condition (approximately 3.2 cases per million people/year), which usually occurs in adults and mainly in women [16]. The most common cause of endogenous hypercortisolism is a pituitary tumor secreting ACTH (Cushing's disease). Small-cell lung cancer is the most common source of ectopic ACTH secretion [17].

Cushing's syndrome is a debilitating disease, lethal if untreated (death rate is 51% at 5 years) [18]. Most common causes of death are infections, cerebrovascular accidents, pulmonary emboli, and myocardial infarction [18]. A complex mechanism controls glucocorticoid secretion involving the hypothalamus (secreting corticotropin releasing hormone), pituitary (secreting ACTH), and adrenal glands [14]. Clinical features of Cushing's syndrome include truncal obesity and limb muscle wasting, facial plethora, hirsutism, menstrual disorders, myopathy, striae, acne, psychological symptoms, congestive heart failure, hypertension, and secondary diabetes mellitus [19]. Mild autonomous hypercortisolism without clinical signs of cortisol excess, which is typically discovered in the context of an adrenal incidentaloma—subclinical

Cushing's syndrome—may be associated with hypertension and impaired glucose tolerance (see Sect. 2.4 of this chapter).

Upon clinical suspicion, biochemical investigations are necessary to confirm the diagnosis, after excluding excessive exogenous glucocorticoid exposure in a close collaboration with endocrinology [17]. Initial steps should include more than one of the screening tests:

- Late night salivary cortisol
- Urinary free cortisol
- Overnight dexamethasone suppression test (1 mg)

After confirming the overproduction of cortisol (and the loss of the normal circadian pattern of secretion), ACTH serum levels will indicate the etiology (pituitary or ectopic—ACTH dependent; adrenal—ACTH independent) [20].

For ACTH-dependent hypercortisolism, it is mandatory to distinguish between pituitary and ectopic origin. A high dose dexamethasone suppression test could be conducted, as well as an MRI of the pituitary gland and a chest CT scan [19]. An abdomen CT scan or MRI is necessary in all cases of ACTH-independent hypercortisolism.

The morbidity and mortality associated with Cushing's syndrome justifies that surgical treatment is indicated in the majority of patients, either pituitary (for pituitary adenomas—Cushing's disease) or adrenal [19]. Normalization of cortisol production is the most efficient way to improve and cure hypercortisolism-related comorbidities, despite the possibility that those complications persisting after Cushing's syndrome have been cured [21]. Indications for adrenalectomy in the context of Cushing's syndrome include unilateral adrenal diseases, bilateral macronodular hyperplasia, primary pigmented nodular adrenocortical disease (PPNAD), failure after pituitary surgery, and in some cases of irresectable or metastatic ACTH secreting tumors [22]. Adrenal adenoma is a benign tumor of cortical cells which usually does not exceed 5 cm. Larger lesions suggest carcinoma [14]. The possibility of malignancy must be always present, since adrenocortical carcinoma (ACC) may secrete cortisol, and features of malignancy (invasion, lymph node involvement, distant metas-

tasis) may not be obvious. Malignancy is not an absolute contraindication for laparoscopic or retroperitoneoscopic surgery, but usually an open approach is the best option for those aggressive tumors [14, 22].

Surgical treatment of unilateral adrenal tumors is straightforward using minimally invasive surgery with cure rates of nearly 100%. After adrenalectomy, it is expectable that all patients develop adrenal insufficiency due to contralateral adrenal atrophy caused by the prolonged ACTH suppression. The hypothalamus-pituitary-adrenal axis usually recovers in 18–30 months. Meanwhile, hydrocortisone reposition is mandatory at an initial dose of 12–15 mg/m^2/day [17].

Primary bilateral macronodular hyperplasia (PBMH) is a rare condition that is more common in children. Bilateral adrenalectomy is the standard treatment for PBMH, with a significant advantage over pharmacological therapies, despite the resulting definitive adrenal insufficiency. Since the intrinsic steroidogenic capacity of adenomatous cells in PBMH is limited, unilateral adrenalectomy may be also effective in controlling cortisol rates. In this case, a straight follow-up is mandatory to check for recurrences [17].

For PPNAD, bilateral adrenalectomy is the treatment of choice in bilateral glandular disease. However, selected patients with mild phenotype may benefit from unilateral adrenalectomy or even partial adrenalectomy, as reported by Walz et al. and Iacoboni et al. [23, 24].

Bilateral adrenalectomy is a second-line treatment of Cushing's disease, in patients not suitable for pituitary surgery or after failure of the surgical treatment. As previously mentioned, bilateral adrenalectomy has the advantage of a rapid cortisol reduction, which must be balanced with the need of permanent glucocorticoid and mineralocorticoid reposition [17].

Surgical resection of ACTH secreting tumors may not be possible in all cases because of local invasion or metastatic disease. In that scenario, bilateral adrenalectomy may be necessary for hypercortisolism control [17].

Bilateral adrenalectomy performed to control hypercortisolism in ACTH-dependent Cushing's syndrome achieves clinical remission in more than 95% of cases, and an improvement of health-related quality of life in 82 to 89% of patients. Surgical morbidity and mortality are 18% and 3%, respectively [22]. In Nelson's syndrome, a condition characterized by corticotropic tumor growth that may develop in patients with Cushing's disease after bilateral adrenalectomy, doctors must actively seek and control both a gradually increasing serum ACTH and skin pigmentation [22].

In 1990, the surgical treatment of Cushing's patients was historically associated with non-neglectable rates of morbidity and mortality of 7–13% and 2.3%, respectively [25]. Those rates decreased dramatically with the advent of minimally invasive surgery, which is a safe procedure, either performed by laparoscopy or by retroperitoneoscopy [25]. In a study of 170 patients submitted to retroperitoneoscopic adrenalectomy (13 bilateral) for Cushing's syndrome, Alesina, a member of the Essen pioneer group headed by Martin Walz, reported no mortality or major morbidity, and an incidence of minor complications of 5.3%. Mean operative time was 53 ± 36 minutes and 99.4% of patients were cured. Only 10% of the patients needed Intensive Care Unit (ICU) support in postoperative period. Operative time and morbidity compare favorably with laparoscopic approach [25]. Retroperitoneoscopic adrenalectomy has another important advantage over laparoscopic surgery—the possibility of simultaneous bilateral surgery, with two surgical teams working at the same time, without patient mobilization, thus reducing operative time [25].

As the laparoscopic approach has made adrenalectomy for Cushing's syndrome a safer therapeutic option, the new possibilities provided by PRA may represent a further improvement in the treatment of this pathology.

2.2.3 Excessive Production of Catecholamines: Pheochromocytoma and Paraganglioma

A pheochromocytoma is a tumor arising from adrenomedullary chromaffin cells that commonly produce one or more catecholamines: epinephrine, norepinephrine, and dopamine. These tumors are rarely biochemically silent [26]. A paraganglioma is a tumor derived from extra-adrenal chromaffin cells of the sympathetic paravertebral ganglia of thorax, abdomen, and pelvis. Paragangliomas can also arise from parasympathetic ganglia located along the glossopharyngeal and vagal nerves in the neck and at the base of the skull [26]. About 80–85% of chromaffin-cell tumors are pheochromocytomas, whereas 15–20% are paragangliomas [26].

The pheochromocytoma was first described in 1886 by Felix Frankel and owes its name to Ludwig Pick in view of its staining with chromium salt: dusky (phaios) color (chroma) [27, 28]. Pheochromocytoma and paraganglioma (PPGL) are rare tumors, with annual incidence of 1–300,000 habitants in the United States, representing 0.2 to 0.6% of the adults with hypertension and 1.7% of hypertensive children, there not being a difference in terms of gender, and a mean age at diagnosis of 55 years in sporadic cases. Hereditary pheochromocytomas are usually diagnosed earlier in life [29]. Pheochromocytomas represent 5% of the incidentally discovered adrenal masses [29]. Pheochromocytomas may occur sporadically or as part of hereditary syndrome. According to the latest studies among patients with non-syndromic pheochromocytoma, up to 24% of tumors may be hereditary, which challenges the ancient 10% rule of pheochromocytoma (10% malignant, 10% bilateral, and 10% extra-adrenal) [30].

Hereditary pheochromocytoma is associated with multiple endocrine neoplasia type 2 (MEN-2A or MEN-2B), neurofibromatosis type 1 (NF-1), von Hippel-Lindau (VHL) syndrome, and familial paragangliomas and pheochromocytomas due to germline mutations of genes encoding succinate dehydrogenase subunits B, C, and D (SDHB, SDHC, SDHD). In general, the traits are inherited in an autosomal dominant pattern [30]. Hereditary pheochromocytomas and paragangliomas have major probability of being bilateral, multifocal, extra-adrenal, or malignant [26]. Malignancy is defined by local invasion or distant metastasis. Tumor size larger than 5 cm, lymphovascular or capsular invasion, and increased Ki67 proliferation index are associated with an increased risk of malignancy [26].

Excessive secretion of catecholamines has noxious effects on the organism leading to an important increase in morbidity and mortality in non-treated patients [26]. PPGL patients can be symptomatic or asymptomatic. Main signs and symptoms of catecholamine excess include hypertension (sustained or episodic), which occurs in more than 90% of the cases, palpitations, headache, sweating, and pallor. Presentation depends on the predominant catecholamine secreted: tumors secreting noradrenaline tend to cause sustained hypertension, whereas tumors secreting adrenaline and noradrenaline often cause episodic hypertension. Only rarely do dopamine secreting tumors cause hypotension [30]. Less common signs and symptoms include fatigue, nausea, weight loss, constipation, flushing, and fever [30]. According to the degree of catecholamine excess, patients may suffer myocardial infarction, arrhythmia, stroke, or other vascular presentations (e.g., any organ ischemia). Similar signs and symptoms are produced by numerous other clinical conditions and, therefore, pheochromocytoma is often referred to as the "great mimic" [30].

Diagnosis of PPGL relies on biochemical evidence of catecholamine production by the tumor. Biochemical testing should be performed in symptomatic patients, patients with an adrenal incidentaloma, and those with a hereditary risk of developing a pheochromocytoma or paraganglioma [30]. Catecholamines are metabolized within chromaffin cells to metanephrines (norepinephrine to normetanephrine and epinephrine to metanephrine, respectively) [26]. Measurements of fractionated metanephrines in urine or plasma provide superior diagnostic sensitivity over measurement of the parent catecholamines [26]. Values four times higher than the upper limit of normal are diagnostic of a functioning pheochromocytoma or paraganglioma. False positive results due to medications, clinical conditions, or inadequate sampling conditions must be excluded. In patients with plasma metanephrine above the upper reference limit but less than four times above that limit, a clonidine suppression test combined with measurements of plasma catecholamines and normetanephrine may prove useful [26].

A positive test must be followed by abdominal imaging since the abdomen is the most probable localization. Both CT and MRI have excellent sensitivity (90–100%) in detecting catecholamine producing tumors with a good specificity (70–80%), especially for tumors >1 cm [26, 30]. Extra-adrenal lesions may occur anywhere along the sympathetic chain and may need investigation with cervical ultrasound, chest-abdomen-pelvis CT, or MRI [26, 30]. Functional imaging uses different methods of nuclear medicine and is indicated for incidental lesions highly suspicious for PPGL with inconclusive biochemical testing, young patients, assessment of regional extension or multifocality, exclusion of metastases and in syndromic disease (MEN 2 A/B, VHL, NF1, SDH-mutation) [26]. These include metaiodobenzylguanidine (MIBG) scan/scintigraphy, positron emission tomography (PET) with 18-fluorodihydroxyphenylalanine (FDOPA), 18-fluorodopamine (FDA), 18-fluorodeoxyglucose (FDG), and PET with radiolabeled dodecane tetraacetic acid (DOTA) peptides [26]. Unequivocal biochemical evidence with typical adrenal imaging does not require functional imaging [26].

In proven evidence of pheochromocytoma and/or paraganglioma, surgical indication is generally given to all patients fit for surgery, due to the cardiovascular morbidity and mortality of uncontrolled catecholamine secretion, as well as to local tumor growth and malignant potential. In metastasized PPGL, surgery aims to prevent local complications, reduce hormone production, and improve successive therapeutic measures [31]. In some metastatic tumors, even debulking of the lesion can help control the symptoms [31]. Due to the high incidence of bilateral adrenal disease in hereditary pheochromocytoma, partial adrenalectomies are advocated in these patients, thereby avoiding morbidity associated with medical adrenal replacement. It remains controversial whether partial adrenalectomies should be considered in patients with a sporadic unilateral pheochromocytoma. However, open surgical approaches could still be necessary in selected patients with locally invasive or malignant disease [30, 31]. The first adrenalectomies for pheochromocytoma were performed in 1926 by Roux, in Lausanne, and by Charles Mayo, in Rochester [32].

Even after the widespread dissemination of laparoscopic adrenalectomy, minimally invasive surgery for pheochromocytoma was met with some reservation due to concerns of adverse hemodynamic sequelae resulting from pneumoperitoneum and gland manipulation, as well as due to the technical challenges involved in removing these highly vascular and generally large tumors [33]. However, after several studies, minimally invasive approach for pheochromocytoma was deemed safe, effective, and resulting in decreased postoperative pain and shorter hospital stays when compared with open adrenalectomy [33]. Open surgical approaches could still be necessary in selected patients with locally invasive or malignant disease. Most position statements also recommended an open approach for tumors >6 cm, ensuring complete tumor resection, preventing tumor rupture, and avoiding local recurrence [31]. As abdominal paragangliomas have more propensity to be malignant, most authors recommend the open approach, but a minimally invasive approach can be performed for small, noninvasive paragangliomas in surgically favorable locations [31].

Current recommendations for patients undergoing surgery for PPGL suggest preoperative α-blockage to prevent perioperative hypertensive crisis. In selective cases with no hypertension or cardiovascular risk factors, preoperative blockage may be omitted [31]. Phenoxybenzamine (α-adrenoceptor blocker) is commonly used for preoperative control of blood pressure (10–20 mg twice daily for 10–14 days). Alternatives to phenoxybenzamine for preoperative blockade include calcium channel blockers and selective competitive α1-adrenoceptor blocking agents, such as terazosin and doxazosin, which have shorter half-lives and lower the risk for postoperative hypotension. A β-adrenoceptor blocker may be used for preoperative control of tachyarrhythmias or angina. However, loss of β-adrenoceptor-mediated vasodilatation in a patient with unopposed catecholamine-induced vasoconstriction can result in dangerous increases in blood pressure. Therefore, β-adrenoceptor blockers should never be employed without first blocking α-adrenoceptor-mediated vasoconstriction [26]. Volume contraction associated with chronic vasoconstriction may occur in patients with PPGL. Recent works by Groeben et al., from the Essen group, suggest that preoperative blockage may not be necessary and can even be associated with an increased rate of complications [34, 35]. Saline infusion or increased water intake is recommended to expand volume and reduce postoperative hypotension [26].

There are no data regarding any difference in recurrence rate after open vs minimally invasive adrenalectomy. Mortality rate is about 1%, and the conversion rate and transfusion rate are about 5% (rate of conversion to open is influenced by tumor size and surgeon experience). Because pheochromocytomas are rare, a prospective randomized study comparing open with minimally invasive surgery is unlikely [26].

When performing a partial adrenalectomy, it is necessary to preserve 1/3 of the gland to maintain sufficient cortical function. Adrenal vein preservation is not necessary if this amount of normal adrenal is kept [27]. Alesina et al., in a series of 66 patients with bilateral pheochromocytomas treated by retroperitoneoscopic cortical-sparing adrenalectomy (32 synchronous surgeries), reported a cortisol-free postoperative course in 60 patients (91%), with one persistence disease needing reoperation, and no recurrences or mortality. Those results confirm the efficacy of retroperitoneoscopic adrenalectomy in the treatment of this disease [27].

A potential advantage of the retroperitoneoscopic approach (RA) over the transperitoneal laparoscopic approach (TLA) in bilateral adrenalectomy is the possibility of resecting both left and right glands simultaneously, as there is no need to change the patient's positioning, which shortens operative time. Studies comparing TLAdr with PRA for pheochromocytoma have concluded that both are safe and effective approaches. However, PRA results in decreased operative times, less blood loss, and lower post-operative length of stay [36]. RA is also suitable for children and adolescents with pheochromocytomas or retroperitoneal paraganglioma, as reported by Walz et al. in a series of 42 patients [36].

2.3 Posterior Retroperitoneoscopic Adrenalectomy in Adrenal Malignancies

2.3.1 Adrenocortical Carcinoma

Adrenocortical carcinoma (ACC) is a rare tumor affecting 1 to 2 patients per million inhabitants, representing 0.2% of all cancer deaths in the United States [37, 38]. In Southern Brazil, the incidence during childhood is 2.9 to 4.2 per million per year, compared with an estimated incidence of 0.2 to 0.3 per million children per year worldwide, which can be mainly attributed to the high prevalence of the p.R337H low-penetrance allele of *TP53* [37]. There are two peaks of increased incidence: in childhood and at 50–55 years, with a slight prevalence in females (ratio female/male ranges from 1.5–2.5:1) [37].

In 2% to 10% of ACC patients, a contralateral tumor is present, either representing a synchronous or a metachronous ACC, making it difficult to determine whether the contralateral tumor is an independent primary tumor or a metastasis to the contralateral gland [37].

Some data suggest a genetic predisposition [37]. Germline *TP53* mutations are the underlying genetic cause of ACC in 50% to 80% of children with ACC [37]. Childhood ACC is a core malignancy of Li–Fraumeni Syndrome (LFS). Other core cancers are choroid plexus tumors, sarcomas, early-onset breast cancers, brain cancers, and leukemias [38]. Because of the impact of a diagnosis of LFS for the patient and at-risk relatives, *TP53* germline testing should be considered in all ACC patients [37]. ACC patients usually present one of three scenarios [37]:

- symptoms and signs of hormone excess (40–60%)
- nonspecific symptoms due to local tumor growth, such as abdominal or flank pain, abdominal fullness, or early satiety (30%)
- incidental finding (20–30%)

Hypercortisolism is the most common presentation in patients with hormone excess (50%–80% of hormone-secreting ACCs), causing the classic signs and symptoms of plethora, muscle weakness/atrophy, diabetes mellitus, and osteoporosis. It is also common that high cortisol levels in ACC saturate the renal HSD11B2 system, resulting in glucocorticoid-mediated mineralocorticoid receptor activation. Therefore, hypokalemia and hypertension are commonly observed in ACC patients with hypercortisolism. When combined with pronounced muscle weakness, these symptoms of rapidly progressive Cushing's syndrome are generally indicative of a malignant adrenal tumor [37]. The second most produced hormones in patients with ACC are adrenal androgens (40–60% of hormone-secreting ACCs), causing rapid-onset male pattern baldness, hirsutism, virilization, and menstrual irregularities in women. Concurrent androgen and cortisol production is frequent (half of hormone-secreting ACC) [37]. Estrogen production occurs in 1–3% of male ACC patients, causing gynecomastia and testicular atrophy (through suppression of the gonadal axis) [37]. Autonomous aldosterone secretion is rare in ACC [37]. At the time of presentation, ACCs are frequently large tumors, measuring on average 10 to 13 cm. Only a minority of tumors are <6 cm (9–14%), with only 3% presenting as lesions <4 cm [37].

The European Network for the Study of Adrenal Tumors (ENSAT) defined a staging system for ACC that became widely adopted [39]. The ENSAT staging system defines 4 stages. Stage 1 (≤5 cm) and stage 2 (>5 cm) tumors are confined to the adrenal gland. Stage 3 tumors extend into surrounding tissue (para-adrenal adipose tissue or adjacent organs) or involve locoregional lymph nodes. Stage 4 is reserved for patients with distant metastasis [39]. Data from more than 400 patients collected by the Michigan Endocrine Oncology Repository reported the following mean stage at diagnosis: stage 1, 14%; stage 2, 45%; stage 3, 27%; and stage 4, 24%. The most common metastatic sites are lung (40–80%), liver (40–90%), and bone (5–20%) [37].

Initial evaluation upon diagnosis must include a physical examination and patient clinical history with particular emphasis on symptoms and signs of hormone excess. A focus on family history is important to identify possible hereditary contributions [37, 40]. A basic biochemical evaluation, which includes creatinine, liver function tests, and a complete blood count should also be performed, as these values may guide further therapy and disease management [31]. The initial hormonal evaluation is essential and must include a dexamethasone suppression test, cortisol levels, 24-hour urine free cortisol, ACTH, dehydroepiandrosterone sulfate (DHEAS), testosterone, aldosterone, renin, metanephrine, and normetanephrine [31, 37]. Patients who have lesions with features suspected of malignancy, as well as patients with signs and symptoms suggestive of sex hormone excess, should have estradiol, DHEAS, and testosterone levels measured [31, 37]. Staging should also include a CT or an MRI of the abdomen and pelvis, and a chest CT scan. Other imaging should be guided by clinical suspicion (e.g., bone scan for skeletal metastasis) [31, 37].

Though ACC prognosis is poor, there is a marked individual variation in disease progression, recurrence, and overall survival. Even in patients with stage 4 disease, survival ranges from a few months to several years [31, 37, 38]. Nowadays, the only curative therapeutic for ACC is complete tumor resection. Adjuvant therapies aim only to decrease the chance of recurrence and all therapy of unresectable or metastatic ACC must be considered palliative [31, 38].

Appropriate preoperative evaluation, operative planning, and a surgical team experienced in adrenal resections are essential to achieve the best outcomes [37]. Unfortunately, most patients with ACC are operated outside reference centers and global results may reflect this lack of expertise [37]. After a thorough medical evaluation,

nearly 25% of stage 3 tumors were preoperatively underestimated as stage 2 [37]. Surgery for stage 4 should be individually decided [31, 37].

Patients with distant metastatic disease in multiple organs, and patients with non-resectable multiple metastatic deposits in one organ, should not be submitted to adrenalectomy [31, 38]. Other options must be considered, such as external beam radiation for palliation, with other adjuncts to improve local symptoms, and better control hormone excess. A tumor thrombus within the vena cava is not a contraindication for surgery if the tumor is otherwise technically resectable [38–40]. Debulking for control of hormone excess in the setting of known metastatic disease can also be performed in some situations, after balancing risks and benefits of an aggressive procedure in a usually debilitated patient [37]. The extension and role of lymph node dissection in ACC remain controversial [31, 37, 38]. In one retrospective study, locoregional lymph node dissection improved tumor staging ability and led to a more favorable oncological outcome in patients with otherwise localized ACC [37]. In adrenal tumors, the main lymphatic areas that should be removed as part of the *en bloc* resection include the renal hilum and the origin of the celiac and mesenteric artery. A balance between the risk caused by the extended surgery and the benefit of radical lymph node dissection must be carefully evaluated on an individual basis. Large prospective studies on this topic are still lacking [31, 37].

The possibility of removing ACC by laparoscopic or retroperitoneoscopic approach is largely debatable (see Chap. 5), and most guidelines recommend an open access [31, 38]. The advantages of a minimally invasive adrenal surgery (lower morbidity, less pain, shorter hospital stays, and decreased overall time to recovery) lose relevance when treating an aggressive tumor like ACC, in which case the initial surgery has strong impact on prognosis. The higher propensity for shedding of malignant cells caused by the laparoscopic instruments, the lack of tactile sensation, and the need for a big incision for removing ACC tumors (usually large) are arguments against minimally invasive surgery in this context [38]. Published data comparing the efficacy of the laparoscopic approach (LA) vs. the open approach (OA) for ACC are limited. All large series are retrospective, include fewer than 200 patients (most reports including fewer than 10 patients), provide limited or no follow-up, and evidence several biases [37, 38]. Considering the available data, the American Association of Clinical Endocrinologists and the American Association of Endocrine Surgeons advocate OA by an experienced surgeon as the procedure of choice, raising the important question of defining what an "experienced" surgeon is [41]. The European Society of Endocrine Surgeons and European Society for Medical Oncology have a more liberal position, suggesting that LA could be performed for stage 1 and 2 ACC tumors less than 8 or 10 cm if an R0 resection is performed and the surrounding periadrenal tissue is removed [37, 40, 42, 43]. More studies are needed to evaluate the possibility and results of lymph node dissection by a minimally invasive approach to treat an ACC.

2.3.2 Malignant Pheochromocytoma and Paraganglioma

Approximately 10% of pheochromocytomas and 15% to 35% of paragangliomas are malignant, with malignancy being defined as the presence of distant metastasis. There are no reliable histological features allowing a distinction between a benign tumor and a malignant primary tumor. Despite local tissue invasion, blood vessel invasion, tumor size larger than 5 cm, and DNA ploidy suggest malignancy, these characteristics do not distinguish between benign and malignant tumors with certainty [44–46]. Efforts are ongoing to identify predictors of malignancy, but only the presence of distant metastases, including locoregional lymph nodes, is widely accepted as a malignant criterion. Metastasis is defined as the appearance of chromaffin tissue in non-chromaffin sites distant from the primary tumor [45]. Metastases occur most frequently in lymph nodes, bone (50%), liver (50%), and lungs (30%)

and can appear as many as 20 years after initial presentation. Liver involvement may be the result of direct continuous spread of the primary tumor [44, 45]. Clinically, there is no significant difference between benign and malignant disease [46].

There is no curative treatment for metastatic pheochromocytoma. Although data suggesting improved survival after surgical debulking is scarce, surgical intervention is favored for palliation of local complications due to metastatic disease and reduction of chromaffin tissue and hormonal activity. Surgical debulking may also be used to increase the efficacy of other therapeutic modalities, but there is no evidence that this therapeutic approach prolongs survival of patients with metastatic disease [44, 45]. The prognosis of malignant pheochromocytoma is poor. Though long-term survival is possible, the overall 5-year survival is less than 50%. Medical control of the catecholamine excess is mandatory. Surgery, radiation therapy or chemotherapy, and new targeted therapies may provide palliative benefit [44–46]. In contrast to benign pheochromocytomas, in which minimally invasive surgery is gold standard, malignant pheochromocytomas often feature large tumors or extra-adrenal tumors in locations difficult to be removed by laparoscopy or retroperitoneoscopy. Therefore, in cases of proven or suspected malignancy, open surgery is recommended. Minimally invasive approaches can eventually be indicated on an individual basis and in centers with large expertise [31].

2.3.3 Metastases to the Adrenal Glands

Metastases to the adrenal glands are the second most common type of adrenal masses after adenomas. Data from the autopsy of patients with malignancies revealed metastases to the adrenal glands in 10–27% of cases. This incidence may be explained by the rich sinusoidal blood flow and the multiple pathways of arterial blood supply to the adrenal glands [47]. Isolated adrenal metastases are rare, most of which are found in patients with disseminated cancer [47].

The increasing survival of cancer patients and the growing use of imaging technology has led to an increment in the number of adrenal metastases found [48]. Lung (39%) and breast (35%) cancers account for most adrenal metastases, but metastases from melanoma, renal cancer, hepatocarcinoma, and colorectal cancer are also frequent [31, 47]. Relative prevalence varies according to geographic region [47].

Isolated adrenal metastasis can be synchronous (discovered at the time of the primary cancer or within 6 months after identification of the primary tumor) or metachronous (found after a disease-free interval [DFI] of more than 6 months). Bilateral adrenal metastases are common [47].

Most patients (95%) with adrenal metastases are asymptomatic at the time of diagnosis [47]. In cases of bilateral metastases to the adrenal glands, symptomatic hormonal insufficiency may develop and should be treated with substitution doses of glucocorticoids before and after adrenalectomy [47]. In case of suspicion of adrenal metastases, it is paramount to rule out gland dysfunction, as up to 48% of adrenal masses in patients with a known malignancy may be true incidentalomas. Ruling out pheochromocytoma is mandatory, as stated in a previous section, but also exclusion of hypercortisolism and hyperaldosteronism must be performed [31].

Imaging investigation must include not only CT or MRI, exams that frequently provide the initial suspicion, but also a PET scan (usually PET/CT) to access further metastatic disease [47, 48]. The suspicion of adrenal metastases is one of the few indications for biopsy of the gland, judiciously reserved for cases in which the doubt persists after noninvasive imaging techniques [38, 48].

Even though the existence of adrenal metastases represents advanced disease with a generally poor prognosis, surgical resection may increase survival, and even cure some patients with a 5-year survival rate of 20–45% [47]. Indications for surgical resection of the adrenal must fulfill the following conditions [47]:

- Control of extra-adrenal disease can be accomplished.

- Metastatic disease only to the adrenal gland(s).
- Adrenal imaging is highly suggestive of metastasis, or the patient has a biopsy-proven adrenal malignancy.
- Metastasis is confined to the adrenal gland as assessed by a recent imaging study.
- The patient's performance status warrants an aggressive approach.

Traditionally, open adrenalectomy was the preferred option for patients with adrenal metastasis, but enhanced experience in minimally invasive techniques has changed this. Solitary adrenal metastases from an extra-adrenal primary neoplasm are generally small and confined to the adrenal gland, making the laparoscopic or retroperitoneoscopic approaches amenable for these cases [31, 47]. The main concern is whether laparoscopic or retroperitoneoscopic adrenalectomy can be considered equivalent to open adrenalectomy from an oncological point of view (recurrence rates and survival time). The proper patient selection remains key in deciding the best treatment. Ensuring wide surgical margins with *en bloc* excision of periadrenal fat is an absolute requirement [47]. There are few studies (only case series) comparing open with minimally invasive adrenalectomy for adrenal metastases. In those studies, no superiority could be attributed to one approach. Additionally, they supported the known advantages of laparoscopy/retroperitoneoscopy in terms of lower blood loss, operative time, hospital stay, and complication rates [47]. The majority of authors report no port-site metastases or locoregional recurrences after minimally invasive adrenalectomy for metastatic tumors, even after a long-term follow-up [47]. Open surgery is perhaps more indicated when preoperative imaging suggests local invasion, large metastases (>9 cm), vena cava thrombus, or significant lymphadenopathies [31].

Studies comparing TLAdr with PRA for adrenal metastases are lacking. Significant adhesions from prior surgery could preclude the TLA. The RA has the advantage of not being affected by prior surgery adhesions, since there is no incursion into the peritoneal cavity. Relative contraindications for the minimally invasive approach include morbid obesity, coagulopathy, and severe cardiopulmonary disease which precludes the hypercapnia associated with pneumoperitoneum/pneumoretroperitoneum [47].

2.4   Adrenal Incidentaloma

The growing utilization of imaging exams allied with the continuous enhancement in image definition has led to the increased discovery of unexpected pathological findings, with variable clinical implications. One of the most common unexpected findings revealed by CT, MRI, or ultrasonography is an incidental adrenal mass or incidentaloma. It is defined as a clinically unapparent adrenal mass > 1 cm in diameter detected during imaging performed for reasons other than for suspected adrenal disease [49, 50]. The overall incidence of adrenal incidentalomas is 4% of the general population, increasing to 7% in patients over 70 years old [50]. Many adrenal incidentalomas, while picked up incidentally, may have clinical symptoms or associated signs on closer questioning and clinical examination, namely those associated with obesity, diabetes mellitus, and hypertension [49]. The finding of an adrenal incidentaloma must be followed by a diagnosis workup directed at answering some pertinent questions [31]:

- Is the mass hormonally active?
- Does the tumor exhibit radiological features of malignancy?
- Does the patient have a personal or familial history of cancer?

Investigation for excessive hormone production, as stated in previous sections, must include a dexamethasone suppression test to exclude adrenal Cushing's syndrome, determination of free metanephrines in plasma and urine to exclude a pheochromocytoma and, in hypertensive patients, the determination of the aldosterone–renin ratio to exclude Conn's syndrome. If the imaging reveals any suspicion of ACC, DHEAS, 17-OH-progesteron, and estradiol should be determined in serum [31].

Although most adrenal incidentalomas are unilateral, bilateral incidentalomas are found in 10–15% of the cases. The most common causes of bilateral adrenal incidentalomas are metastases, PBMH, and bilateral cortical adenomas. Other causes of bilateral incidentalomas include bilateral pheochromocytomas, congenital adrenal hyperplasia, Cushing's disease, or ectopic ACTH secretion with secondary bilateral adrenal hyperplasia [50]. Up to 15% of patients with an adrenal incidentaloma will have a hormonally active tumor [31, 50].

A tumor >6 cm has a malignancy risk of 25%. Additionally, vascular invasion, lack of well-demarcated margins, and presence of suspicious lymph nodes are also radiological features suggestive of malignancy [31, 49, 50]. A CT with adrenal protocol and measurement of the Hounsfield Units (HU) is useful to distinguish between benign and malignant tumors. A threshold value of 10 HU has a sensitivity of 71% and a specificity of 91% for benignity. Incidentalomas with >10 HU attenuation require more detailed evaluation [31, 50]. Familial or personal history of cancer must raise the suspicion of adrenal metastases. In a patient without a past medical history of malignancy, the probability of an adrenal nodule being malignant is very low. On the contrary, for a patient with known cancer, this probability is considerably higher, with metastases occurring in 32–72% of these cases [47]. For surgical treatment of adrenal metastases, see Chap. 5 and previous section of current chapter (2.3.3 Metastases to the Adrenal Glands).

Surgery for adrenal incidentalomas is indicated in functioning nodules, or in nodules ≥6 cm, excluding myelolipoma, which usually does not indicate resection [31, 39, 40]. Nonfunctioning adrenal tumors <4 cm, which carry a low risk of malignancy (< 2%), do not usually indicate resection [31, 39]. There is no consensus for adrenal tumors between 4 and 6 cm without radiological features of malignancy. A tailored approach, either surveillance or minimally invasive adrenalectomy, must be discussed with the patient [31, 39]. For tumors <6 cm without suspicion of malignancy, a minimally invasive approach is recommended [49]. Larger tumors can also be amenable to transperitoneal laparoscopic or retroperitoneoscopic resection, depending on the surgeon's expertise [31].

In many cases of adrenal incidentalomas with documented autonomous cortisol hypersecretion (ACS), cortisol secretion rates may not be significantly elevated. As a result, the patient may be asymptomatic, has no clinical features, and has few comorbidities that may be ascribed to cortisol hypersecretion. ACS is defined as an alteration of the hypothalamic-pituitary-adrenal axis, characterized by ACTH-independent cortisol excess, often without clinical signs and symptoms of overt Cushing's syndrome [31]. In the past, terms as "subclinical Cushing's syndrome," "subclinical hypercortisolism," and "preclinical Cushing's syndrome" have all been used to describe this condition [31]. Despite the absence of signs and symptoms, ACS has been associated with hypertension, insulin resistance, type 2 diabetes mellitus, obesity, metabolic syndrome, and increased mortality. ACS is the commonest functional abnormality in patients with adrenal incidentalomas, with a prevalence of up to 20% [50]. Indication for surgery must be tailored to the patient with ACS, taking into consideration that metabolic improvement after adrenalectomy, including weight loss, blood pressure-lowering, glucose tolerance, lower lipids, and beneficial effects on bone have been reported [50]. A recent systematic review addressed the cardiovascular benefit of surgery in ACS patients. The adrenalectomy improves cardiovascular outcomes and mortality in these patients [50]. This decision must also balance the severity of clinical features against the risks of surgery in an aged population, whose comorbidities could be coincidentally age-related and without causative relation to a false positive ACS diagnosis, leading to unnecessary surgery [50].

Follow-up of non-operated adrenal incidentalomas is not consensual. The American Association of Clinical Endocrinologists recommends repeating the imaging for up to 5 years for benign tumors, whereas the European Guidelines do not recommend further imaging for benign, nonfunctioning lesions with less than 4 cm. Patients with adrenal lesions over 4 cm or inde-

terminate lesions who have not undergone surgery are recommended to repeat imaging in 6 to 12 months. The optimal timing depends on the index of suspicion [39, 41, 50]. Surgical resection is recommended if there is a 20% increase in size, in addition to at least a 5 mm increase in diameter over the same period. Both adrenocortical cancers and metastases usually demonstrate rapid growth over months, in contrast to a benign adenoma. Further imaging should be undertaken once again at 6–12 months [39, 41, 50].

Repeating hormonal testing is not advised in patients without evidence of hormone oversecretion on their initial assessment. It should only be considered if patients develop new clinical signs and symptoms of adrenal hormone hypersecretion or in case of worsening of comorbidities, including diabetes, hypertension, or osteoporosis [50].

Patients with ACS have a low risk of progressing to overt Cushing's syndrome, but since ACS is associated with numerous comorbidities, patients not initially operated on must be reassessed annually for cortisol hypersecretion and potential worsening of comorbidities. If there is clinical or biochemical progression, then patients can be re-evaluated for surgery [50].

2.5 Partial Adrenalectomy

Partial (or subtotal) adrenalectomy or cortex preserving adrenalectomy was first proposed by Irvin et al., in 1983, for the treatment of hereditary bilateral pheochromocytoma aiming at preserving the adrenocortical function and avoiding lifelong steroid replacement therapy [50]. In 1995, Walz et al. presented the first cases of retroperitoneoscopic partial adrenalectomies [51].

Nowadays, indications for partial adrenalectomy include not only bilateral adrenal masses, but also solitary masses in context of hereditary diseases with increased risk of developing multiple adrenal tumors [27, 32, 36]. Usually, nonfunctional adrenal tumors have no indication for partial adrenalectomy, since their formal surgical indication is the suspicion of malignancy, which makes total adrenalectomy mandatory [31].

There is a trend towards the use of partial adrenalectomy in the treatment of small adrenal masses. In the future, minimally invasive partial adrenalectomy may become the standard treatment of small benign and functioning adrenal tumors [50].

There is no need to preserve the adrenal vein to warrant adrenal cortical function if a minimum of 1/3 of the gland is kept in place and there is no excessive and unnecessary dissection. This allows for an adequate vascular supply and blood drainage of the adrenal remnant by the diaphragmatic and retroperitoneal collateral arteries and veins, respectively [27]. In the pheochromocytoma, the adrenal vein should be divided to prevent hypertensive crisis due to the discharge of catecholamines secreted by the medulla into the venous system [36]. The use of intraoperative ultrasound can be helpful in tumor localization to preclude unnecessary dissection [36, 50].

References

1. Alemanno G, Bergamini C, Prosperi P, Valeri A. Adrenalectomy: indications and options for treatment. Updat Surg. 2017;69(2):119–25.
2. Gagner M, Lacroix A, Prinz RA, Bolté E, Albala D, Potvin C, et al. Early experience with laparoscopic approach for adrenalectomy. Surgery. 1993;114(6):1120–4.
3. Walz MK, Peitgen K, Hoermann R, Giebler RM, Mann K, Eigler FW. Posterior retroperitoneoscopy as a new minimally invasive approach for adrenalectomy: results of 30 adrenalectomies in 27 patients. World J Surg. 1996;20(7):769–74.
4. Walz MK, Alesina PF, Wenger FA, Deligiannis A, Szuczik E, Petersenn S, at. Posterior retroperitoneoscopic adrenalectomy-results of 560 procedures in 520 patients. Surgery. 2006;140(6):943–8.
5. Perrier ND, Kennamer DL, Bao R, Jimenez C, Grubbs EG, Lee JE, et al. Posterior retroperitoneoscopic adrenalectomy: preferred technique for removal of benign tumors and isolated metastases. Ann Surg. 2008;248(4):666–74.
6. Hundemer GL, Vaidya A. Primary Aldosteronism diagnosis and management: a clinical approach. Endocrinol Metab Clin N Am. 2019;48(4):681–700.
7. Funder JW, Carey RM, Mantero F, Murad MH, Reincke M, Shibata H, et al. The Management of Primary Aldosteronism: case detection, diagnosis, and treatment. An Endocrine Society clinical practice guideline. J Clin Endocrinol Metab. 2016;101(5):1889–916.
8. Conn JW, Presidential address. I. Painting background. II. Primary aldosteronism, a new clinical syndrome. J Lab Clin Med. 1955;45(1):3–17.
9. Lee FT, Elaraj D. Evaluation and Management of Primary Hyperaldosteronism. Surg Clin North Am. 2019;99(4):731–45.
10. Zhou Y, Zhang M, Ke S, Liu L. Hypertension outcomes of adrenalectomy in patients with primary aldosteronism: a systematic review and meta-analysis. BMC Endocr Disord. 2017;17(1):61.
11. Young WF. Diagnosis and treatment of primary aldosteronism: practical clinical perspectives. J Intern Med. 2019;285(2):126–48.
12. Waldmann J, Maurer L, Holler J, Kann PH, Ramaswamy A, Bartsch DK, et al. Outcome of surgery for primary hyperaldosteronism. World J Surg. 2011;35(11):2422–7.
13. Gavriilidis P, Camenzuli C, Paspala A, Di Marco AN, Palazzo FF. Posterior Retroperitoneoscopic versus laparoscopic Transperitoneal adrenalectomy: a systematic review by an updated meta-analysis. World J Surg. 2021;45(1):168–79.
14. Norton JA, Li M, Gillary J, Le HN. Cushing's syndrome. Curr Probl Surg. 2001;38(7):488–545.
15. Arnaldi G, Angeli A, Atkinson AB, Bertagna X, Cavagnini F, Chrousos GP, et al. Diagnosis and complications of Cushing's syndrome: a consensus statement. J Clin Endocrinol Metabol. 2003;88(12):5593–602.
16. Wengander S, Trimpou P, Papakokkinou E, Ragnarsson O. The incidence of endogenous Cushing's syndrome in the modern era. Clin Endocrinol. 2019;91(2):263–70.
17. Nieman LK, Biller BM, Findling JW, Murad MH, Newell-Price J, Savage MO, et al. Treatment of Cushing's syndrome: an Endocrine Society clinical practice guideline. J Clin Endocrinol Metab. 2015;100(8):2807–31.
18. Clayton RN. Mortality in Cushing's disease. Neuroendocrinology. 2010;92(1):71–6.
19. Nieman LK. Diagnosis of Cushing's syndrome in the modern era. Endocrinol Metab Clin N Am. 2018;47(2):259–73.
20. Fleseriu M, Auchus R, Bancos I, Ben-Shlomo A, Bertherat J, Biermasz NR, et al. Consensus on diagnosis and management of Cushing's disease: a guideline update. Lancet Diabetes Endocrinol. 2021;9(12):847–75.
21. Ferriere A, Tabarin A. Cushing's syndrome: treatment and new therapeutic approaches. Best Pract Res Clin Endocrinol Metab. 2020;34(2):101381.
22. Di Dalmazi G, Reincke M. Adrenal surgery for Cushing's syndrome: an update. Endocrinol Metab Clin N Am. 2018;47(2):385–94.
23. Iacobone M, Albiger N, Scaroni C, Mantero F, Fassina A, Viel G, et al. The role of unilateral adrenalectomy in ACTH-independent macronodular adrenal hyperplasia (AIMAH). World J Surg. 2008;32(5):882–9.
24. Walz MK, Peitgen K, Diesing D, Petersenn S, Janssen OE, Philipp T, et al. Partial versus total adrenalec-

tomy by the posterior retroperitoneoscopic approach: early and long-term results of 325 consecutive procedures in primary adrenal neoplasias. World J Surg. 2004;28(12):1323–9.

25. Alesina PF, Hommeltenberg S, Meier B, Petersenn S, Lahner H, Schmid KW, et al. Posterior retroperitoneoscopic adrenalectomy for clinical and subclinical Cushing's syndrome. World J Surg. 2010;34(6):1391–7.

26. Lenders JW, Duh QY, Eisenhofer G, Gimenez-Roqueplo AP, Grebe SK, Murad MH, et al. Pheochromocytoma and paraganglioma: an endocrine society clinical practice guideline. J Clin Endocrinol Metab. 2014;99(6):1915–42.

27. Alesina PF, Hinrichs J, Meier B, Schmid KW, Neumann HP, Walz MK. Minimally invasive cortical-sparing surgery for bilateral pheochromocytomas. Langenbeck's Arch Surg. 2012;397(2):233–8.

28. Welbourn RB. Early surgical history of phaeochromocytoma. Br J Surg. 1987;74(7):594–6.

29. Jain A, Baracco R, Kapur G. Pheochromocytoma and paraganglioma - an update on diagnosis, evaluation, and management. Pediatr Nephrol. 2020;35(4):581–94.

30. Chen H, Sippel RS, O'Dorisio MS, Vinik AI, Lloyd RV, Pacak K. The north American neuroendocrine tumor society consensus guideline for the diagnosis and management of neuroendocrine tumors: pheochromocytoma, paraganglioma, and medullary thyroid cancer. Pancreas. 2010;39(6):775–83.

31. Lorenz K, Langer P, Niederle B, Alesina P, Holzer K, Nies C, et al. Surgical therapy of adrenal tumors: guidelines from the German Association of Endocrine Surgeons (CAEK). Langenbeck's Arch Surg. 2019;404(4):385–401.

32. Uludağ M, Aygün N, İşgör A. Surgical indications and techniques for adrenalectomy. Sisli Etfal Hastan Tip Bul. 2020;54(1):8–22.

33. Dickson PV, Alex GC, Grubbs EG, Ayala-Ramirez M, Jimenez C, Evans DB, et al. Posterior retroperitoneoscopic adrenalectomy is a safe and effective alternative to transabdominal laparoscopic adrenalectomy for pheochromocytoma. Surgery. 2011;150(3):452–8.

34. Groeben H, Nottebaum BJ, Alesina PF, Traut A, Neumann HP, Walz MK. Perioperative α-receptor blockade in phaeochromocytoma surgery: an observational case series. Br J Anaesth. 2017;118(2):182–9.

35. Groeben H, Walz MK, Nottebaum BJ, Alesina PF, Greenwald A, Schumann R, et al. International multicentre review of perioperative management and outcome for catecholamine-producing tumours. Br J Surg. 2020;107(2):e170–8.

36. Walz MK, Iova LD, Deimel J, Neumann HPH, Bausch B, Zschiedrich S, et al. Minimally invasive surgery (MIS) in children and adolescents with Pheochromocytomas and retroperitoneal Paragangliomas: experiences in 42 patients. World J Surg. 2018;42(4):1024–30.

37. Else T, Kim AC, Sabolch A, Raymond VM, Kandathil A, Caoili EM, et al. Adrenocortical carcinoma. Endocr Rev. 2014;35(2):282–326.

38. Kiernan CM, Lee JE. Minimally invasive surgery for primary and metastatic adrenal malignancy. Surg Oncol Clin N Am. 2019;28(2):309–26.

39. Fassnacht M, Arlt W, Bancos I, Dralle H, Newell-Price J, Sahdev A, et al. Management of adrenal incidentalomas: European Society of Endocrinology Clinical Practice Guideline in collaboration with the European network for the study of adrenal tumors. Eur J Endocrinol. 2016;175(2):G1–g34.

40. Fassnacht M, Dekkers OM, Else T, Baudin E, Berruti A, de Krijger R, et al. European Society of Endocrinology Clinical Practice Guidelines on the management of adrenocortical carcinoma in adults, in collaboration with the European network for the study of adrenal tumors. Eur J Endocrinol. 2018;179(4):g1–g46.

41. Zeiger MA, Thompson GB, Duh QY, Hamrahian AH, Angelos P, Elaraj D, et al. The American Association of Clinical Endocrinologists and American Association of endocrine surgeons medical guidelines for the Management of Adrenal Incidentalomas. Endocr Pract. 2009;15(Suppl 1):1–20.

42. Henry JF, Peix JL, Kraimps JL. Positional statement of the European Society of Endocrine Surgeons (ESES) on malignant adrenal tumors. Langenbeck's Arch Surg. 2012;397(2):145–6.

43. Berruti A, Baudin E, Gelderblom H, Haak HR, Porpiglia F, Fassnacht M, et al. Adrenal cancer: ESMO clinical practice guidelines for diagnosis, treatment and follow-up. Ann Oncol. 2012;23 Suppl 7:vii131–8.

44. Harari A, Inabnet WB 3rd. Malignant pheochromocytoma: a review. Am J Surg. 2011;201(5):700–8.

45. Adjallé R, Plouin PF, Pacak K, Lehnert H. Treatment of malignant pheochromocytoma. Horm Metab Res. 2009;41(9):687–96.

46. Gimm O, DeMicco C, Perren A, Giammarile F, Walz MK, Brunaud L. Malignant pheochromocytomas and paragangliomas: a diagnostic challenge. Langenbeck's Arch Surg. 2012;397(2):155–77.

47. Sancho JJ, Triponez F, Montet X, Sitges-Serra A. Surgical management of adrenal metastases. Langenbeck's Arch Surg. 2012;397(2):179–94.

48. Serra C. Metástases Suprarrenais Revista Portuguesa de Cirurgia. 2015;32:27–34.

49. Lee JM, Kim MK, Ko SH, Koh JM, Kim BY, Kim SW, et al. Clinical guidelines for the Management of Adrenal Incidentaloma. Endocrinol Metab (Seoul). 2017;32(2):200–18.

50. Sherlock M, Scarsbrook A, Abbas A, Fraser S, Limumpornpetch P, Dineen R, et al. Adrenal Incidentaloma. Endocr Rev. 2020;41(6):775–820.

51. Walz MK, Peitgen K, Krause U, Eigler FW. Dorsal retroperitoneoscopic adrenalectomy-a new surgical technique. Zentralbl Chir. 1995;120(1):53–8.

Open Versus Minimally Invasive Approach

3

Hugo Louro and Jaime Vilaça

3.1 Introduction

The first laparoscopic adrenal resection was performed by Michel Gagner in 1992 [1]. Soon after, several groups published their series of cases enhancing the advantages of this new approach that includes shorter postoperative hospital length of stay (HLOS), less wound complications, reduced pain, and a faster return to normal daily activities [2–4].

3.2 Validation of Laparoscopic Adrenal Surgery

The aforementioned advantages set the tone for surgeons to study the feasibility and efficacy of laparoscopic adrenalectomy after the Gagner et al. report. The sum of the most relevant of these works is detailed in Table 3.1. Although most of them are retrospective studies and were conducted with a relatively small number of patients, the advantage of the laparoscopic approach for well-selected cases is clear. Laparoscopic adrenalectomy is better than the open approach in what concerns intraoperative blood loss, HLOS, and overall complications. The operative times tend to be longer in the laparoscopic adrenalectomy. However, when surgical teams gained experience in advanced laparoscopic techniques (particularly adrenalectomy), the operative times were comparable to the open approach in some works [2, 4]. Also, fewer postoperative analgesics and a faster return to regular activity were pointed out as important advantages of laparoscopic adrenalectomy when compared to the open approach [3–7]. Therefore, as with many abdominal surgeries, laparoscopy is considered the gold standard for adrenal surgery in most patients.

H. Louro (✉)
General Surgery, Centro Hospitalar Vila Nova de Gaia/Espinho, Vila Nova de Gaia, Portugal

J. Vilaça
General Surgery, Hospital da Luz, Porto, University of Minho, Braga, Porto, Portugal

© The Author(s), under exclusive license to Springer Nature Switzerland AG 2023
C. E. Costa Almeida (ed.), *Posterior Retroperitoneoscopic Adrenalectomy*,
https://doi.org/10.1007/978-3-031-19995-0_3

27

Table 3.1 Worldwide publications comparing open surgery with laparoscopic approach for adrenal surgery

Study (Year)	No of procedures	Type of Approach (LA vs OA)	Design	No of centers	Length of study (years)	Tumor size (cm) LA	Tumor size (cm) OA	Operating time (min) LA	Operating time (min) OA	Blood loss (ml) LA	Blood loss (ml) OA	HLOS (days) LA	HLOS (days) OA	Complications % LA	Complications % OA
Prinz [5] (1995)	34	10 vs. 11 vs. 13[a]	Retrospective	1	N/A	4.8 ± 1.8 (8/3)	5.1 ± 2.1 (8/1) 3.1 ± 1.6 (7/1.5)[a]	212 ± 77 (341/90)	174 ± 41 (275/137) 139 ± 36 (212/80)[a]	228 ± 66 (700/100)	391 ± 88 (700/150) 288 ± 118 (500/200)[a]	2.1 ± 0.9 (4/1)	6.4 ± 1.5 (8/4) 5.5 ± 2.9 (13/3)[a]	N/A	N/A
MacGillivray[6] (1996)	29	17 vs. 12	Retrospective	1	4.5	N/A	N/A	289 ± 86	201 ± 108	198 (144)	500 (574)	7.9 ± 4.9	1 ± 1.6	21	56
Staren [7] (1996)	43	21 vs. 22	Retrospective	1	5	3.2 (8/1)	9.2 (25/2)	206 (241/90)	177 (299/137)	N/A	N/A	2.2 (7/1)	6.1 (8/4)	N/A	N/A
Linos [8] (1997)	165	18 vs. 86 vs. 61[a]	Retrospective	1[b]	11	4 (6.5/2)	8 (20/2.5) 5.3 (14/0.5)[a]	116 (180/75)	155 (315/75) 109 (160/95)[a]	N/A	N/A	2.3 (5/1)	8 (25/2) 4.5 (11/1)[a]	0	6 (6/7)[a]
Jacobs [4] (1997)	38	19 vs. 19	Retrospective	1	6	2.5 ± 1.2	3.3 ± 1.9	164 ± 107	151 ± 63	109 ± 75	263 ± 242	2.3 ± 0.9	5.1 ± 1.7	3	16
Thompson [9] (1997)	100	50 vs. 50[a]	Retrospective	1	4	2.9	2.9	167	127	N/A	N/A	3.1	5.7	6	54
Vargas [10] (1997)	40	20 vs. 20	Retrospective	2	4	13.9 ± 6	11.5 ± 4	193 ± 14	178 ± 17	245 ± 52	283 ± 62	3.1 ± 0.3	7.2 ± 0.6	10	25
Dudley [2] (1999)	53	31 vs. 22[a]	Retrospective	2	8	4.1 (8.2/1)	2.9 (5/1)	158 (315/90)[c]	85 (110/60)[c]	175 (500/0)	350 (2000–100)	3.5 (5/2)	8.5 (11/6)	6	55
Imai [11] (1999)	80	40 vs. 40	Retrospective	1	7	2.8 ± 1.7	2.7 ± 1.4	180	127	40	162	12	18	5	50
Shen [12] (1999)	80	42 vs. 38	Retrospective	1	23	N/A	N/A	N/A	N/A	N/A	N/A	N/A	N/A	0	11
Ichikawa [3] (2000)	74	38 vs. 36	Retrospective	1	8	2.3 ± 1 (5.2/0.8)	2.6 ± 1.1 (4.5/1)	225 ± 89 (480/85)	122 ± 39 (230/65)	138 ± 186 (720/5)	188 ± 200 (862/14)	8.5 ± 3.7 (20/4)	12.9 ± 3.5 (28/9)	8	6
Hazzan [13] (2001)	54	28 vs. 28	Retrospective	1	3	3.6 (8/0.5)	2.9 (7/0.5)	188	139	N/A	N/A	4	7.5	16	39
Ortega [14] (2002)	20	10 vs. 10	Retrospective	1	4	N/A	N/A	110 ± 29	123 ± 30	N/A	N/A	3.7 ± 1.2	5.8 ± 1.6	10	20

LA laparoscopic approach, *OA* open approach, *N/A* not available

The values of tumor size, operating time, blood loss, and HLOS represent the mean ± standard deviation or mean (maximum/minimum)

[a]Posterior approach

[b]All adrenalectomies performed by the same surgeon

[c]Unilateral adrenalectomies

3.3   Still a Place for Open

Thirty years have passed since the first report of laparoscopic adrenal resection and there is a stronghold for open surgery in this domain. As in the endoscopic approach, open surgery can use the anterior and posterior route to reach the retroperitoneal adrenal gland.

This chapter summarizes existing comparative studies and reviews current indications for different open approaches.

3.4   Open Surgery

3.4.1   Current Indications

Besides the lack of laparoscopic expertise in a specific center that for whatever reason cannot transfer its patients, there are still clear indications for the open approach. Laparoscopy should be used in this domain mostly for benign pathology. Malignant adrenal tumors, namely adrenal carcinoma, tend to be very fragile and therefore, the violation of their integrity with the consequent spread of the disease can be disastrous. Additionally, the involvement of neighboring structures or extreme size can make laparoscopy very difficult or even impossible. Thus, it is now consensual that suspicion of malignancy, size greater than 12 cm, and contiguous invasion of adjacent structures are formal indications for open surgery. Malignant pheochromocytoma is better performed open, and for small metastatic disease laparoscopy can be considered (see Chapters 2 and 5). Apart from indication, general aspects such as heart failure, coagulopathy, or severe respiratory dysfunction may preclude laparoscopy [15, 16]. Indications for open adrenalectomy are summarized in Table 3.2.

Table 3.2 Indications for open adrenalectomy

Tumors >12 cm
Malignancy
Coagulopathy
Cardiopulmonary high-risk patients

3.4.2   Risk of Conversion to Open

Conversion to open is a rare event ($\approx$5%), but should be considered under these circumstances: detected intraoperative local invasion; detected regional lymph node metastasis; inability to remove the tumor completely (without spillage); inability to laparoscopically control an intraoperative complication [17]. Of course, the best way is to prevent the need for reactive conversion.

In the opinion of some researchers, obesity can increase the risk of conversion [16, 18, 19]. Tumor size should be judged by the surgical team sparingly because the greater the risk of malignancy, the greater the risk of conversion in inverse proportion to the surgeon's experience. The large size of the tumor is related to an obvious difficulty due to subverted anatomy, increased surface of dissection, and narrow "working" space [16, 20]. Despite this, new devices such as endo-staplers or advanced energy coagulation have made it easier to perform laparoscopically in these more difficult cases.

Another point frequently highlighted by some authors is the risk of conversion due to previous abdominal surgeries. Although this condition can be considered as a relative contra-indication for transabdominal approach, conversion is rarely attributed to this factor [15]. In a large series of 865 patients, previous abdominal surgery did not predict the need of conversion [19]. Finally, it is imperative to consider surgical team experience, hospital volume, and a multidisciplinary approach to these patients in order to reduce either the risk of conversion or the upfront indication for open adrenalectomy due to tumor size.

3.5   Open Technique

Although it falls outside the scope of this book, the conventional technique of open surgery is succinctly described. As in laparoscopic surgery, anterior (laparotomy) and posterior (lumbotomy) approaches are considered. For *en bloc* resection of very large masses, sometimes locally advanced tumors, a thoracoabdominal incision should be considered.

The first surgery of the adrenal glands was carried out in 1889, when Scottish surgeon John Knowsley-Thornton performed a large left adrenal tumor excision on a 35-year-old female patient. Only in the 1920s would the first adrenalectomies for pheochromocytoma be performed in Europe by César Roux (Lausanne, Switzerland), and in the United States by Charles Mayo (Rochester, Minnesota). The first adrenal resections were made through a midline abdominal incision. Charles Mayo would describe it from the flank and Young, from a posterior incision (Baltimore, Maryland) [17].

The most common approach is the transperitoneal anterior for an open procedure. The posterior approach avoids abdominal adhesions related to previous laparotomy and can also reduce wound complications that are more frequent in obese patients and in those with Cushing's syndrome. Due to small working space, this approach is rarely used for tumors above 6 cm. The lateral extraperitoneal approach is also a good option for obese patients.

3.5.1 Anterior Approach

Usually, the main indication for open anterior adrenalectomy is the suspicion of cancer or proven malignancy. Within this scope, the technique presented respects this assumption.

3.5.1.1 Technique for the Right Side

The patient is placed in supine position and a wide, right subcostal incision is made, which may be extended to the left side, depending on the size of the tumor. As shown in Fig. 3.1, several incisions may be used in the anterior approach. However, a wide subcostal incision allows for a better ribs retraction, improved liver mobilization, providing optimal access to the adrenal gland, kidney, and inferior vena cava (IVC).

When in the peritoneal cavity, the entire abdomen should be inspected for deposits of malignant disease. The use of intraoperative ultrasound can be useful in locoregional assessment of the disease, namely in the involvement of adrenal vein, IVC, and the existence of a malignant thrombus [21]. The first step is to proceed to the mobilization of the liver, rotating the right hepatic lobe medially, which allows for complete IVC exposure from the base of the thorax to the renal hilum. If the invasion of the liver is identified, a rim of normal liver should be resected *en bloc* with the specimen [21, 22].

The right adrenal vein is then identified and ligated in a standard fashion. All the fat medial to the adrenal gland, as well as lymph nodes posterior to the renal hilum and in the inter-aorto-cava space should be retrieved. An optimal IVC exposure should be achieved, allowing

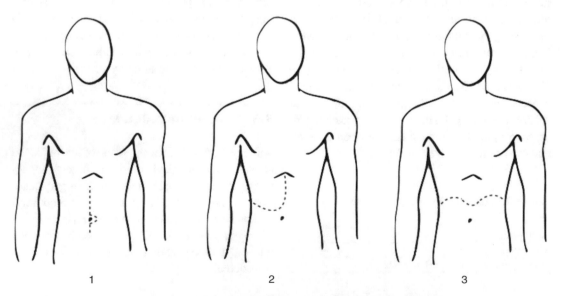

Fig. 3.1 Anterior transperitoneal approach. (1) Midline incision; (2) Makuuchi modified incision; (3) Bilateral subcostal transverse incision

a cavotomy and thrombectomy in case of tumoral thrombus [21]. The dissection is extended inferiorly until the superior half of the kidney, excising any fat around the kidney and the posterior peritoneal lining to obtain a clean inferior margin.

The next step consists in dissecting the adrenal gland from the kidney's upper pole, proceeding posteriorly and laterally, excising all retroperitoneal fat around the tumor, and exposing the posterior musculature. Finally, dissection continues superiorly, reaching the diaphragm, completing the tumor's resection. After excision of the specimen, metal clips can be placed to mark the tumor bed for eventual adjuvant radiotherapy.

3.5.1.2 Technique for the Left Side
The left open adrenalectomy occurs in a similar fashion to the right adrenalectomy. It begins with the patient in supine position and a wide left subcostal incision, which may be extended to the right side.

After the systematic inspection of the peritoneal cavity, the splenic flexure of the colon is mobilized following a wide incision through the white line of Toldt. Then, the phreno-splenic ligament is divided, allowing spleen and pancreatic tail retraction, exposing the left adrenal gland, the kidney, and the aorta. At this point, one must be careful not to cause any injury to the splenic hilum [22].

The left renal vein is carefully dissected, and the adrenal vein identified and ligated. Dissection progresses medially with ligation of arterial branches coming from the aorta. The posterior limit of dissection is the posterior musculature that extends superiorly until the left diaphragmatic crus [22, 23]. When performing dissection of the plan between the left adrenal gland and the kidney, one should be aware of a possible superior renal artery which, in case of injury, may cause renal ischemia [22].

The remaining surgery is completed in a similar fashion as for the right adrenalectomy, resecting all the surrounding fat *en bloc* with the gland specimen [21].

3.5.2 Posterior Approach

Considered as the gold standard technique for small and benign adrenal tumors during several years, the posterior adrenalectomy is presented as the most direct route to the gland. This is reflected in several advantages over the open anterior approach, namely less blood loss, lower HLOS, and less overall mortality [24]. However, the surgical field is narrow and access to the adrenal vein and great vessels is suboptimal, which could be a problem, particularly in an excessive bleeding scenario [23]. As previously mentioned, this technique is usually limited to tumors smaller than 6 cm in diameter.

The patient is placed in a prone position and an angled incision is made from medial to lateral over the 12th rib, as shown in Fig. 3.2. After division of the subcutaneous tissue and the latissimus dorsi and sacrospinalis muscles, the 12th rib is exposed and excised. At this point, one should be

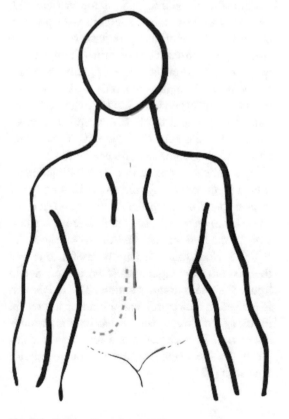

Fig. 3.2 Retroperitoneal approach

careful not to cause injury to the neurovascular bundle.

Once in the retroperitoneum, the kidney is mobilized inferiorly, and the adrenal gland is identified. The plan between the medial border of the gland and IVC is dissected, and the adrenal vein is identified and ligated in a standard manner. In the case of the left adrenalectomy, the dissection is made between medial border of the gland and the aorta, and the adrenal vein runs a longer course, usually draining into the left renal vein.

3.5.3 Thoracoabdominal Approach

The open adrenalectomy via thoracoabdominal approach is usually reserved for large, right-sided tumors with marked involvement of the surrounding structures and the IVC, since it allows the best exposure of the retroperitoneum, adrenal gland, and major vessels [22, 23]. This approach is associated with a heavy burden of postoperative problems such as incisional pain, phrenic nerve injury, and pulmonary complications which eventually require a chest tube. For this reason, it is generally reserved for large right-sided tumors, in which both the liver and the IVC can limit the exposure, and a safe control of the IVC in the upper part of the abdomen may be needed.

The patient is placed in a semi-oblique position, with the operating side upwards. A body roll is positioned at the patient's waist to open the angle between the ribs and the iliac crest. An incision is made over the 8th/9th rib as shown in Fig. 3.3. Sometimes, it may be useful to excise the rib, but the surgeon must be careful not to injure the neurovascular bundle. The diaphragm is incised in a circumferential manner to prevent injury to the phrenic nerve, entering the abdominal cavity. The adrenal gland resection is completed in the same way as the open anterior approach [23].

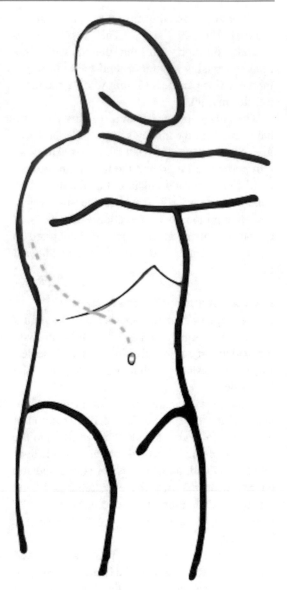

Fig. 3.3 Thoracoabdominal approach

3.6 Conclusion

Although most adrenal surgery cases are now approached laparoscopically, specific indications for conventional open surgery remain. Not only should the endocrine surgeon master these approaches, but the cases proposed for adrenalectomy must be presented and discussed by a multidisciplinary team that includes surgery, radiology, anesthesiology, and endocrinology in order to establish the best surgical approach.

References

1. Gagner M, Lacroix A, Prinz RA, Bolté E, Albala D, Potvin C, et al. Early experience with laparoscopic approach for adrenalectomy. Surgery. 1993;114(6):1120–4. discussion 1124–5.
2. Dudley NE, Harrison BJ. Comparison of open posterior versus transperitoneal laparoscopic adrenalectomy. Br J Surg. 1999;86(5):656–60.
3. Ichikawa T, Mikami K, Komiya A, Suzuki H, Shimizu A, Akakura K, et al. Laparoscopic adrenalectomy for functioning adrenal tumors: clinical experiences with 38 cases and comparison with open adrenalectomy. Biomed Pharmacother. 2000;54(Suppl 1):178s–82s.
4. Jacobs JK, Goldstein RE, Geer RJ. Laparoscopic adrenalectomy. A new standard of care. Ann Surg. 1997;225(5):495–501. discussion 501–2
5. Prinz RA. A comparison of laparoscopic and open adrenalectomies. Arch Surg. 1995;130(5):489–92. discussion 492–4
6. MacGillivray DC, Shichman SJ, Ferrer FA, Malchoff CD. A comparison of open vs laparoscopic adrenalectomy. Surg Endosc. 1996;10(10):987–90.
7. Staren ED, Prinz RA. Adrenalectomy in the era of laparoscopy. Surgery. 1996;120(4):706–9. discussion 710–1
8. Linos DA, Stylopoulos N, Boukis M, Souvatzoglou A, Raptis S, Papadimitriou J. Anterior, posterior, or laparoscopic approach for the management of adrenal diseases? Am J Surg. 1997;173(2):120–5.
9. Thompson GB, Grant CS, van Heerden JA, Schlinkert RT, Young WF Jr, Farley DR, et al. Laparoscopic versus open posterior adrenalectomy: a case-control study of 100 patients. Surgery. 1997;122(6):1132–6.
10. Vargas HI, Kavoussi LR, Bartlett DL, Wagner JR, Venzon DJ, Fraker DL, et al. Laparoscopic adrenalectomy: a new standard of care. Urology. 1997;49(5):673–8.
11. Imai T, Kikumori T, Ohiwa M, Mase T, Funahashi H. A case-controlled study of laparoscopic compared with open lateral adrenalectomy. Am J Surg. 1999;178(1):50–3. discussion 54
12. Shen WT, Lim RC, Siperstein AE, Clark OH, Schecter WP, Hunt TK, et al. Laparoscopic vs open adrenalectomy for the treatment of primary hyperaldosteronism. Arch Surg. 1999;134(6):628–31. discussion 631–2
13. Hazzan D, Shiloni E, Golijanin D, Jurim O, Gross D, Reissman P. Laparoscopic vs open adrenalectomy for benign adrenal neoplasm. Surg Endosc. 2001;15(11):1356–8.
14. Ortega J, Sala C, Garcia S, Lledo S. Cost-effectiveness of laparoscopic vs open adrenalectomy: small savings in an expensive process. J Laparoendosc Adv Surg Tech A. 2002;12(1):1–5.
15. Assalia A, Gagner M. Laparoscopic adrenalectomy. Br J Surg. 2004;91(10):1259–74.
16. Alemanno G, Bergamini C, Prosperi P, Valeri A. Adrenalectomy: indications and options for treatment. Updat Surg. 2017;69(2):119 25.
17. Uludag M, Aygun N, Isgor A. Surgical indications and techniques for adrenalectomy. Sisli Etfal Hastan Tip Bul. 2020;54(1):8–22.
18. Shen ZJ, Chen SW, Wang S, Jin XD, Chen J, Zhu Y, et al. Predictive factors for open conversion of laparoscopic adrenalectomy: a 13-year review of 456 cases. J Endourol. 2007;21(11):1333–7.
19. Vidal O, Saavedra-Perez D, Martos JM, de la Quintana A, Rodriguez JI, Villar J, et al. Risk factors for open conversion of lateral transperitoneal laparoscopic adrenalectomy: retrospective cohort study of the Spanish adrenal surgery group (SASG). Surg Endosc. 2020;34(8):3690–5.
20. Taffurelli G, Ricci C, Casadei R, Selva S, Minni F. Open adrenalectomy in the era of laparoscopic surgery: a review. Updat Surg. 2017;69(2):135–43.
21. Miller BS. Management of Adrenal Cortical Tumors. In: Cameron JL, Cameron AM, editors. Current surgical therapy. 13th ed. Philadelphia, PA: Elsevier; 2019. p. 741–9.
22. Mirallié E, et al. Técnicas quirúrgicas de adrenalectomía. EMC - Urología. 2020;52(1):1–7.
23. Lim SK, Rha KH. Surgery of the adrenal glands. In: Partin AW, Dmochowski RR, Kavoussi LR, Peters C, editors. Campbell-Walsh-Wein urology. 12th ed. Philadelphia, PA: Elsevier; 2020. p. 2405–26.
24. Russell CF, Hamberger B, van Heerden JA, Edis AJ, Ilstrup DM. Adrenalectomy: anterior or posterior approach? Am J Surg. 1982;144(3):322–4.

Retroperitoneoscopic Versus Laparoscopic Adrenalectomy

4

Oscar Vidal, Martí Manyalich Blasi, and David Saavedra-Perez

4.1 Background and Clinical Considerations

Since adrenalectomy was successfully performed for the first time, adrenal surgery has seen great advances, especially in terms of minimally invasive surgery. In the last decades, adrenalectomy has made a breakthrough, which turned a large incision over to a minimally invasive surgery. The first documented successful laparoscopic adrenalectomy (LA) was performed by Michel Gagner and was published in 1992 [1]. Compared with open adrenalectomy, subsequent experience has demonstrated a shift over LA with the main advantages of short hospitalization, low morbidity rate, and earlier return to normal activity [2, 3]. As consequence, LA has become the "gold standard" technique to treat small to medium size benign adrenal tumors [4–6].

There are several LA techniques to remove an adrenal gland. Among the multiple approaches of LA, transperitoneal laparoscopic adrenalectomy (TLAdr) is more popular because most surgeons are more familiar with anatomy and operating view. TLAdr uses a cut through the belly that includes cutting a membrane inside the abdomen (the peritoneum) to expose the adrenal gland. Since TLAdr was proposed in 1992, its surgical indications have been widely increased. At present, the technique is not only considered to be the standard procedure for adrenal tumors less than 6 cm in diameter. Ample data subsequently has demonstrated the suitability of the transperitoneal laparoscopic approach in removing all but the largest adrenal tumors with a reduction in pain and a shortened length of stay without increasing the operating time or morbidity [7–12].

The laparoscopic transperitoneal monopoly in minimally invasive adrenalectomy, however, was broken by Bonjer et al. that demonstrated the effectiveness of the lateral retroperitoneal adrenalectomy for tumors less than 6 cm [13]. However, the extraperitoneal approach failed to gather traction until Walz et al. popularized the alternative posterior retroperitoneoscopic approach (PRA) using the same instrumentation as in TLAdr with the patient in a modified prone position. The Walz approach has since been widely adopted with minimal modifications worldwide as an alternative to TLAdr [14].

O. Vidal · M. M. Blasi (✉) · D. Saavedra-Perez
General & Digestive Surgery Department, ICMDIM, Hospital Clinic Barcelona, IDIBAPS, University of Barcelona, Barcelona, Spain
e-mail: ovidal@clinic.cat;
manyalich@clinic.cat; dsaavedr@clinic.cat

Table 4.1 Comparison of principal advantages and disadvantages of PRA approach vs LTA approach

	Advantages	Disadvantages
Transperitoneal	– Larger surgical field (important in large tumors) – Examination of the entire abdominal cavity – Easier to teach	– Increased risk of incisional hernias – Longer operating time – In case of bilateral adrenalectomy, need to reposition the patient – Potential increase in difficulty in patients with previous abdominal surgeries – Intolerance to pneumoperitoneum
Retroperitoneal	– Less operative time – Less postoperative pain – Greater conservation of aesthetics – In case of bilateral adrenalectomy, no need to reposition the patient	– Intolerance to the prone position – Small surgical field – Potential increase in intraocular pressure in prolonged surgeries

The PRA has been increasingly favored in recent years as an alternative method of adrenal tumors, especially for patients with a history of abdominal surgery because it can directly and rapidly get into the surgical area without mobilizing intraperitoneal organs. Laparoscopic retroperitoneal adrenalectomy approaches the adrenal gland from the back, without cutting the peritoneum. Moreover, PRA has an outstanding advantage, which can accomplish bilateral adrenalectomy without repositioning the patient and has shown its feasibility for adrenal tumors less than 8 cm in diameter [15, 16].

However, PRA is not easy for beginners to learn because surgeons are not familiar with this anatomic view of the retroperitoneal space. Despite these several benefits, PRA might pose serious additional technical difficulties such as smaller working space, the requirement for the surgeon to learn a new anatomic perspective, and the uncomforting to work with tumors larger than 8 cm [17]. Also, the need of a dedicated staff to know all the nuances of the patient position, equipment, and anesthesia in prone decubitus must be considered.

In tertiary high-volume centers, both mainstream minimal access adrenalectomy procedures can safely be applied in appropriately selected patients. Analyzing the literature, TLAdr and PRA were found to be similar in terms of intra- and postoperative complications and demonstrated clinically equivalent outcomes [18–20]. However, advocates of the latter technique (PRA) have proposed better results. As reported recently,

thanks to the avoidance of pneumoperitoneum and the direct approach to the gland leading to minimal dissection of body wall or adjacent organs, PRA has several advantages such as shorter operative time, lower postoperative pain, and shorter hospitalization with comparable morbidity rate. Mortality rate is approaching 0% in both techniques [18, 19, 21].

Reports of good intra- and postoperative outcomes of PRA have made this method more popular. Nevertheless, up to present, the final choice between RPA or TLAdr remains influenced by surgeon's preference [22]. The most relevant features of PRA and TLAdr approach are resumed in Table 4.1.

4.2   Intraoperative Outcomes

In terms of operation time, the literature reflects a shorter operation time in PRA approach compared to TLAdr, and it is consistent with most studies [19, 23]. The shorter operation time in PRA is most likely due to the smaller extent of dissection required. Other factors such as previous abdominal surgery and tumor laterality might also be expected to impact upon this, particularly in TLAdr, due to the presence of adhesions in the peritoneal cavity and the need to mobilize the liver/spleen. In fact, one of the most important advantages of PRA is the direct approach to the adrenal gland and vein, avoiding the need to enter the peritoneal cavity or mobilize adjacent intraabdominal organs, as well as obviating adhesions from previous surgery, leading to a great saving of time. For this reason, PRA is feasible and ideal also for patients who underwent a previous laparotomy [21]. In addition, in case of bilateral adrenalectomies, the prone position allows to approach both adrenal glands without the need to reposition the patient and sometimes two surgical staff might perform two operations at the same time [21, 24]. In the other hand, surgeon and institutional volume are consistently shown to be important factors impacting in the outcome of endocrine surgical patients and adrenalectomy is no exception.

It is reported in the literature significant difference in respect of operation time because the surgeon has lack of experience in PRA remarking the importance for surgeons to reach proficiency [25–27]. Moreover, when PRA is performed by surgeons skilled in the laparoscopic technique for TLAdr, allowing them to overcome the learning curve for PRA more easily, due to the smaller extent of dissection required, median operative time become shorter for PRA than TLAdr. A comparison of the first 50 operations performed by the developers of PRA and 50 operations performed by a surgical team that learned PRA from the developers found that the learning curve was shorter in the latter group, suggesting that comprehensive training resulted in a shorter operation time and a lower conversion rate. Hence, PRA is safe when performed by surgeons with TLAdr experience or those who undergo proper PRA training [20, 28, 29]. The Walz group also has shown that despite a flattening of the learning curve after 30–40 TLAdr and PRA, relative improvements in operative time are seen even after 500 operations [30].

Several demographic features have previously been reported as impacting on intraoperative parameters of TLAdr and PRA such as operative time and conversion rates. A BMI (Body Mass Index) ≥ 30 kg/m^2 has been shown to be associated with a prolonged operative time in TLAdr. The male gender is also associated with increased operative time, perhaps because of the increased visceral and perinephric fat in men compared to women. Obesity is retained an important and spreading risk factor affecting morbidity also

after TLAdr. It is reported in the literature a positive correlation between BMI and operating time, postoperative complications, and hospitalization as the result of a suboptimal visualization in the context of increased amount of intraperitoneal fat [25, 27, 28, 31]. PRA is also difficult to perform in patients with tumors larger than 7–8 cm and in patients with a high BMI [30].

After the establishment of the PRA beyond the learning curve also is demonstrated that PRA has significantly less estimated blood loss (EBL) than TLAdr, as it is the surgeon and institutional volume, observing a reduction in EBL and operative time with operative volume [18, 32, 33].

In a sense, the studies describe that patient which undergoes PRA suffers less tissue damage during the operation and has a faster recovery after surgery, which may be caused by anatomic structure and gas pressure. The significant difference in EBL is possibly caused by relatively less dissection during PRA. As is known to all, the less the anatomical separation, the relative reduction in blood loss. Also, the lower EBL in the PRA group may reflect the use of this approach for smaller tumors or may be a result of the technique presenting fewer opportunities for blood loss from viscera such as the liver and spleen. The elevated pressure required in PRA to gain the working space (usually 18–25 mmHg) and subsequent tamponade of minor bleeding from small vessels produced by the closed space, preventing greater blood loss may also be a factor. Meanwhile, the high retroperitoneal insufflation pressure usually could lead to compress the inferior vena cava (IVC) or renal vein, reduce venous returns from the adrenal gland and ultimately reduce intraoperative blood loss [34].

The conversion rate is around 2–14% in patients who underwent PRA, while 1–22% in TLAdr patients, with no statistically significant difference but the reasons for conversion differed [18, 28]. The main causes for conversion during TLAdr are bleeding, followed by intra-abdominal adhesions, failure to progress, splenic and pancreatic injury and IVC injury or infiltration, whereas indications for conversion in PRA patients include failure to progress and mainly is associated with inadequate preparation of the retroperitoneal working space or loss of pneumoret-roperitoneum due to surgeon inexperience [28, 33, 35, 36]. Although concerns have been raised regarding the high CO_2 pressure required for PRA, there are no significant complications associated with high pressure [37].

4.3   Postoperative Outcomes

The hospital length of stay (HLOS) after surgery is an important indicator to evaluate the postoperative recovery. In addition, shorter HLOS also mean less hospitalization medical expenses of the patients and relatively higher turnover rate in the hospitals.

As reported in the literature, there is a statistically significant reduction in HLOS in PRA compared to TLAdr. The HLOS of the patients who underwent PRA is generally shorter than the TLAdr patients (1 vs 2–3 days) as described by many authors [38, 39]. The superiority of PRA may be due to the location of the adrenal glands in the posterior aspect of the retroperitoneum and the avoidance of pneumoperitoneum. PRA directly approaches this space, enabling adrenalectomy without collateral damage to adjacent intra-abdominal organs, which must be dissected and mobilized during TLAdr or open adrenalectomy. In consequence, recovery of bowel movement is faster and postoperative ileus is rarely observed in the patients who underwent PRA.

Also, shorter hospital stay might be associated with the reduction of postoperative pain as suggested by the median visual analog scale (VAS) pain score value in patients undergoing PRA than TLAdr. The intensity of postoperative pain and/or nausea has been an important factor associated with early or delayed hospital discharge. Most of the patients who do not present pain or nausea are discharged home on the next day after surgery, and only those that show high VAS scores for these symptoms stayed longer. Postoperative pain and/or nausea delays the onset of oral intake and mobilization, and consequently the HLOS. Patients operated by retroperitoneal approach might show less intensity of these postoperative symptoms mainly due to the preservation of the peritoneal layer. Entering the peritoneum triggers a higher response for pain and nausea and consequently a longer postoperative hospitalization.

Another parameter indicating the amount of postoperative pain is analgesic use during hospitalization, which is lower after PRA in many studies. As interesting data, a study reported that 60% of patients who underwent PRA required no narcotic analgesia, were mobilized, and started the diet on the evening of surgery, demonstrating a faster recovery of bowel movements [21, 29, 31, 38].

The unique complication associated only with PRA is neuromuscular pain related to subcostal nerve injury. The subcostal nerve passes below the twelfth rib and the injury to this nerve commonly occurs during open posterior adrenalectomy, leading to chronic incision-related back pain. Likewise, trocar insertion in this area during PRA can cause nerve damage. The incidence of nerve damage in the largest PRA series is reported to be 9% but is temporary in most patients [30, 40, 41].

References

1. Gagner M, Lacroix A, Bolte E. Laparoscopic adrenalectomy in Cushing's syndrome and Pheochromocytoma. N Engl J Med. 1992;327(14):1033. https://doi.org/10.1056/NEJM199210013271417.
2. Tiberio GA, Baiocchi GL, Arru L, Agabiti Rosei C, De Ponti S, Matheis A, et al. Prospective randomized comparison of laparoscopic versus open adrenalectomy for sporadic Pheochromocytoma. Surg Endosc. 2008;22(6):1435–9. https://doi.org/10.1007/s00464-008-9904-1.
3. Conzo G, Pasquali D, Gambardella C, Della Pietra C, Esposito D, Napolitano S, et al. Long-term outcomes of laparoscopic adrenalectomy for Cushing disease. Int J Surg. 2014;12(Suppl 1):s107–11. https://doi.org/10.1016/j.ijsu.2014.05.036.
4. Bonjer HJ, van der Harst E, Steyerberg EW, de Herder WW, Kazemier G, Mohammedamin RS, et al. Retroperitoneal adrenalectomy: open or endoscopic? World J Surg. 1998;22(12):1246–9.
5. Imai T, Kikumori T, Ohiwa M, Mase T, Funahashi H. A case-controlled study of laparoscopic compared with open lateral adrenalectomy. Am J Surg. 1999;178(1):50–3.
6. Thompson GB, Grant CS, van Heerden JA, Schlinkert RT, Young WF Jr, Farley DR, et al. Laparoscopic

versus open posterior adrenalectomy: a case–control study of 100 patients. Surgery. 1997;122(6):1132–6.

7. Tiberio GA, Solaini L, Arru L, Merigo G, Baiocchi GL, Giulini SM. Factors influencing outcomes in laparoscopic adrenal surgery. Langenbeck's Arch Surg. 2013;398(5):735–43.

8. Boylu U, Oommen M, Lee BR, Thomas R. Laparoscopic adrenalectomy for large adrenal masses: pushing the envelope. J Endourol. 2009;23(6):971–5.

9. Zografos GN, Farfaras A, Vasiliadis G, Pappa T, Aggeli C, Vassilatu E, et al. Laparoscopic resection of large adrenal tumors. JSLS. 2010;14(3):364–8.

10. Tsuru N, Suzuki K, Ushiyama T, Ozono S. Laparoscopic adrenalectomy for large adrenal tumors. Endourol. 2005;19(5):537–40.

11. Telem DA, Nguyen SQ, Chin EH, Weber K, Divino CM. Laparoscopic resection of giant adrenal cavernous hemangioma. JSLS. 2009;13(2):260–2.

12. Gagner M, Pomp A, Heniford BT, Pharand D, Lacroix A. Laparoscopic adrenalectomy: lessons learned from 100 consecutive procedures. Ann Surg. 1997;226(3):238–46.

13. Bonjer HJ, Sorm V, Berends FJ, Kazemier G, Steyerberg EW, de Herder WW, et al. Endoscopic retroperitoneal adrenalectomy: lessons learned from 111 consecutive cases. Ann Surg. 2000;232(6):796–803.

14. Walz MK, Peitgen K, Hoermann R, Giebler RM, Mann K, Eigler FW. Posterior retroperitoneoscopy as a new minimally invasive approach for adrenalectomy: results of 30 adrenalectomies in 27 patients. World J Surg. 1996;20(7):769–74.

15. Conzo G, Tartaglia E, Gambardella C, Esposito D, Sciascia V, Mauriello C, et al. Minimally invasive approach for adrenal lesions: systematic review of laparoscopic versus Retroperitoneoscopic adrenalectomy and assessment of risk factors for complications. Int J Surg. 2016;28(Suppl 1):S118–23. https://doi.org/10.1016/j.ijsu.2015.12.042.

16. Kozlowski T, Choromanska B, Wojskowicz P, Astapczyk K, Lukaszewicz J, Rutkowski D, et al. Laparoscopic adrenalectomy: lateral Transperitoneal versus posterior retroperitoneal approach - prospective randomized trial. Wideochir Inne Tech Maloinwazyjne. 2019;14(2):160–9. https://doi.org/10.5114/wiitm.2019.84694.

17. Agha A, Iesalnieks I, Hornung M, Phillip W, Schreyer A, Jung M, et al. Laparoscopic trans- and retroperitoneal adrenal surgery for large tumors. J Minim Access Surg. 2014;10(2):57–61.

18. Constantinides VA, Christakis I, Touska P, Palazzo FF. Systematic review and meta-analysis of retroperitoneoscopic versus laparoscopic adrenalectomy. Br J Surg. 2012;99(12):1639–48.

19. Chai YJ, Won HK, Yu HW, Kim SJ, Choi JY, Lee KE, et al. Systematic review of surgical approaches for adrenal tumors: lateral transperitoneal versus posterior retroperitoneal and laparoscopic versus robotic adrenalectomy. Int J Endocrinol. 2014;2014:918346.

20. Constantinides VA, Christakis I, Touska P, Meeran K, Palazzo F. Retroperitoneoscopic or laparoscopic adrenalectomy? A single-centre UK experience. Surg Endosc. 2013;27(11):4147–52.

21. Cabalag MS, Mann GB, Gorelik A, Miller JA. Comparison of outcomes after laparoscopic versus posterior retroperitoneoscopic adrenalectomy: a pilot study. Surg Laparosc Endosc Percutan Tech. 2014;24(1):62–6.

22. Shen WT, Grogan R, Vriens M, Clark OH, Duh QY. One hundred two patients with pheochromocytoma treated at a single institution since the introduction of laparoscopic adrenalectomy. Arch Surg. 2010;145(9):893–7. https://doi.org/10.1001/archsurg.2010.159.

23. Meng C, Du C, Peng L, Li J, Li J, Li Y, et al. Comparison of posterior retroperitoneoscopic adrenalectomy versus lateral transperitoneal laparoscopic adrenalectomy for adrenal tumors: a systematic review and meta-analysis. Front Oncol. 2021;10(11):667985. https://doi.org/10.3389/fonc.2021.667985.

24. Sommerey S, Foroghi Y, Chiapponi C, Baumbach SF, Hallfeldt KJ, Ladurner R, et al. Laparoscopic adrenalectomy-10- year experience at a teaching hospital. Langenbeck's Arch Surg. 2015;400(3):341–7.

25. Chai YJ, Yu HW, Song RY, Kim SJ, Choi JY, Lee KE. Lateral transperitoneal adrenalectomy versus posterior retroperitoneoscopic adrenalectomy for benign adrenal gland disease: randomized controlled trial at a single tertiary medical center. Ann Surg. 2019;269(5):842–8. https://doi.org/10.1097/SLA.0000000000002603.

26. van Uitert A, d'Ancona FCH, Deinum J, Timmers H, Langenhuijsen JF. Evaluating the learning curve for retroperitoneoscopic adrenalectomy in a high-volume Center for laparoscopic adrenal surgery. Surg Endosc. 2017;31(7):2771–5. https://doi.org/10.1007/s00464-016-5284-0.

27. Alesina PF. Retroperitoneal adrenalectomy – learning curve, practical tips and tricks, what limits its wider uptake. Gland Surg. 2019;8(Suppl 1):S36–40. https://doi.org/10.21037/gs.2019.03.11.

28. Dickson PV, Alex GC, Grubbs EG, Ayala-Ramirez M, Jimenez C, Evan DB, et al. Posterior retroperitoneoscopic adrenalectomy is a safe and effective alternative to transabdominal laparoscopic adrenalectomy for pheochromocytoma. Surgery. 2011;150(3):452–8.

29. Lee CR, Walz MK, Park S, Park JH, Jeong JS, Lee SH, et al. A comparative study of the transperitoneal and posterior retroperitoneal approaches for laparoscopic adrenalectomy for adrenal tumors. Ann Surg Oncol. 2012;19(8):2629–34.

30. Walz MK, Alesina PF, Wenger FA, Deligiannis A, Szuczik E, Petersenn S, et al. Posterior retroperitoneoscopic adrenalectomy – results of 560 procedures in 520 patients. Surgery. 2006;140(6):943–8.

31. Lombardi CP, Raffaelli M, De Crea C, Sollazzi L, Perilli V, Cazzato MT, et al. Endoscopic adrenalectomy: is there an optimal operative approach?

Results of a single-center case-control study. Surgery. 2008;144(6):1008–14. discussion 1014–5

32. Arezzo A, Bullano A, Cochetti G, Cirocchi R, Randolph J, Mearini E, et al. Transperitoneal versus retroperitoneal laparoscopic adrenalectomy for adrenal tumours in adults. Cochrane Database Syst Rev. 2018;12(12):CD011668.

33. Greco F, Hoda MR, Rassweiler J, Fahlenkamp D, Neisius DA, Kutta A, et al. Laparoscopic adrenalectomy in urological centres – the experience of the German laparoscopic working group. BJU Int. 2011;108(10):1646–51.

34. Ban EJ, Yap Z, Kandil E, Lee CR, Kang SW, Lee J, et al. Hemodynamic stability during adrenalectomy for Pheochromocytoma: a case control study of posterior retroperitoneal vs lateral Transperitoneal approaches. Medicine (Baltimore). 2020;99(7):e19104. https://doi.org/10.1097/MD.0000000000019104.

35. Naya Y, Nagata M, Ichikawa T, Amakasu M, Omura M, Nishikawa T, et al. Laparoscopic adrenalectomy: comparison of transperitoneal and retroperitoneal approaches. BJU Int. 2002;90(3):199–204.

36. Ramacciato G, Nigri GR, Petrucciani N, DiSanto V, Piccoli M, Buniva P, et al. Minimally invasive adrenalectomy: a multicenter comparison of transperitoneal and retroperitoneal approaches. Am Surg. 77(4):409–16.

37. Giebler RM, Walz MK, Peitgen K, Scherer RU. Hemodynamic changes after retroperitoneal CO_2 insufflation for posterior retroperitoneoscopic adrenalectomy. Anesth Analg. 1996;82(4):827–31.

38. Kiriakopoulos A, Economopoulos KP, Poulios E, Linos D. Impact of posterior retroperitoneoscopic adrenalectomy in a tertiary care center: a paradigm shift. Surg Endosc. 2011;25(11):3584–9.

39. Schreinemakers JM, Kiela GJ, Valk GD, Vriens MR, Rinkes IH. Retroperitoneal endoscopic adrenalectomy is safe and effective. Br J Surg. 2010;97(11):1667–72.

40. Siperstein AE, Berber E, Engle KL, Duh QY, Clark OH. Laparoscopic posterior adrenalectomy: technical considerations. Arch Surg. 2000;135(8):967–71.

41. Buell JF, Alexander HR, Norton JA, Yu KC, Fraker DL. Bilateral adrenalectomy for Cushing's syndrome: anterior versus posterior surgical approach. Ann Surg. 1997;225(1):63–8.

Retroperitoneoscopic Approach in Malignant Disease

Oscar Vidal, David Saavedra-Perez, and Martí Manyalich Blasi

5.1 Introduction

The number of adrenalectomies performed worldwide has increased, as the performance and quiality of abdominal imaging with identificaction of adrenal nodules has improved [1]. Thus, the rate of adrenalectomy is also increasing [2, 3]. Over the past 30 years, the minimally invasive adrenal surgery (MIAS) has almost replaced open surgery in the management of most adrenal pathologies and tumors [3, 4]. Benefits of MIAS are widely reported, such as decreased blood loss, transfusion requirement, procedure times, hospital stay, and complications when compared with open adrenalectomy [4]. Options for MIAS are the transperitoneal laparoscopic approach (TLA) and the retroperitoneoscopic approach (RA) [4]. Systematic literature reviews and meta-analyses comparing both MIAS approaches have

been reported and summarized in Chap. 4 of this book [4–6]. However, MIAS for malignant disease remains controversial due to the uncertainty regarding oncologic outcomes relative to open adrenalectomy, in particular for primary adrenal malignancy [7–10]. Despite this and the international guidelines recommendations for surgical treatment on adrenal malignancy, the European registry EUROCRINE for adrenal surgery, that included 658 adrenalectomies from 21 European centers, between 2015 and 2019, reported MIAS in 28% of the patients with adrenocortical carcinoma (ACC) and in 66% of those with adrenal metastases with a conversion rate of 20% [3]. This rate of MIAS for malignant adrenal diseases is consistent with previous retrospective, prospective, and meta-analysis reports [4–6]. In this chapter, we review the recommendations for the preoperative evaluation of patients with adrenal tumors to identify and discuss the indications for MIAS with a special emphasis on the retroperitoneoscopic approach for: (1) indeterminate adrenal nodules suspicious for malignancy, (2) metastatic disease, and (3) primary adrenal cancer.

O. Vidal · D. Saavedra-Perez (✉) · M. M. Blasi
General & Digestive Surgery Department, ICMDIM, Hospital Clinic Barcelona, IDIBAPS, University of Barcelona, Barcelona, Spain
e-mail: ovidal@clinic.cat;
dsaavedr@clinic.cat; manyalich@clinic.cat

5.2 Preoperative Evaluation of Patients with Adrenal Lesions Suspicious for Malignancy

The ESMO-EURACAN Clinical Practice Guidelines recommends that all patients with suspected adrenal malignancy should be discussed in a multidisciplinary expert team meeting [11]. Every patient with malignant suspicious adrenal lesion should undergo careful clinical assessment, including case history, clinical examination for signs and symptoms of adrenal hormone excess [11]. The goal of biochemical evaluation is to assess for the presence of hypercortisolism, hyperaldosteronism, or catecholamine excess (Table 5.1) [1, 11].

This evaluation is essential when a malignant primary or metastatic lesion is suspected because identification of a functional mass will affect management [10]. Patients with bilateral adrenal tumors suspected of bilateral adrenal metastases should undergo cortisol and adrenocorticotropic hormone (ACTH) determination to screen for adrenal insufficiency [1, 10]. Two-thirds of ACCs produce and release excess hormones that can affect perioperative management, prognosis, and treatment of recurrent and metastatic disease, and therefore should be evaluated preoperatively [12]. Furthermore, the rate of adrenal metastases in patients with history of cancer with an adrenal mass is 27% to 73% [13, 14]. Thus, before performing a biopsy of an adrenal lesion concerning for metastasis, biochemical evaluation for pheochromocytoma is recommended due to the risk of hypertensive crisis [10].

The two most commonly used imaging modalities in the initial evaluation of patients with adrenal tumors are computed tomography (CT) scan and magnetic resonance imaging (MRI) [1, 11]. In general, malignant adrenal lesions are heterogeneous in appearance with an irregular shape and indistinct margins. ACCs tend to be large (>4 cm) and exhibit rapid growth; in contrast, metastatic lesions can present at a range of different sizes and exhibit variable growth patterns (Table 5.2) [1].

Table 5.1 Biochemical evaluation of an adrenal tumor

Phenotype	Test
Pheochromocytoma	Urine fractionated metanephrines/plasma metanephrines
Hypercortisolism	Dexamethasone suppression test (1 mg): If >3ug/dL or 1.8–3 ug/dL and comorbidities, measure urine free cortisol, dehydroepiandrosterone sulfate, nocturnal cortisol (saliva/plasma), consider dehydroepiandrosterone sulfate
Primary hyperaldosteronism	Aldosterone/renin activity or direct renin ratio
Excess of sex steroids	Testosterone, dehydroepiandrosterone sulfate, estradiol, or estrone if clinical images suggest adrenal carcinoma
Primary adrenal insufficiency	Serum cortisol in patients with bilateral lesions (suspected infiltration or bleeding)
Congenital adrenal hyperplasia	17-OH progesterone in bilateral lesions or hyperplasia

Modified from Araujo-Castro M, Iturregui Guevara M, Calatayud Gutiérrez M, Parra Ramírez P, Gracia Gimeno P, Hanzu FA, Lamas Oliveira C. Practical guide on the initial evaluation, follow-up, and treatment of adrenal incidentalomas Adrenal Diseases Group of the Spanish Society of Endocrinology and Nutrition. Endocrinol Diabetes Nutr (Engl Ed). 2020 Jun-Jul;67(6):408–419 [1].

Primary and metastatic malignant adrenal tumors tend to have increased and persistent contrast accumulation due to neovascularization of the tumor and therefore demonstrate less washout of contrast on delayed imaging [1, 10]. CT is also helpful in providing information regarding local invasion, presence of bilateral or multifocal primary tumors and extra-adrenal metastatic disease [1, 10]. MRI can be helpful, when iodinated contrast is contraindicated or to avoid radiation exposure [1, 10]. Malignant lesions demonstrate enhancement on T2-weighted images [1, 10].

Adrenal biopsy is recommended only in situations in which the results will influence management. For example, to confirm the presence of isolated metastasis to the adrenal gland in a patient with history of malignancy in whom confirmation of it would result in a recommendation

Table 5.2 Radiological features of adrenal malignant tumors

	Feature
Adrenal carcinoma	– Irregular, heterogeneous, >4 cm with calcifications and bleeding – High attenuation in CT (>20HU), heterogeneous enhancement after contrast administration in CT – Delay in contrast washout – MRI: Hypointense T1. Moderate hyperintensity T2 – Elevated SUVmax in PET-FDG
Metastasis	– Irregular, heterogeneous, and often bilateral – High attenuation in CT (>20HU), enhancement after contrast administration in CT – Delay in contrast washout – MRI: Hypointense T1. Moderate hyperintensity T2 – Elevated SUVmax in PET-FDG

PET-FDG fluorodeoxyglucose positron emission tomography, *MRI* magnetic resonance imaging, *CT* computed tomography

Modified from Araujo-Castro M, Iturregui Guevara M, Calatayud Gutiérrez M, Parra Ramírez P, Gracia Gimeno P, Hanzu FA, Lamas Oliveira C. Practical guide on the initial evaluation, follow-up, and treatment of adrenal incidentalomas Adrenal Diseases Group of the Spanish Society of Endocrinology and Nutrition. Endocrinol Diabetes Nutr (Engl Ed). 2020 Jun-Jul;67(6):408–419 [1]

for systemic therapy [1, 10, 11]. Adrenal biopsy should be avoided in lesions concerning for ACC, unless required to initiate systemic therapy (borderline resectable or metastatic ACC) [1, 10, 11].

5.3 Minimally Invasive Adrenal Surgery for Indeterminate Adrenal Nodules Suspicious for Malignancy

An indeterminate adrenal nodule is >4 cm but <6 cm of size, has >1 cm of growth in 1 year, has some imaging feature concerning for malignancy (Table 5.2) or has clinical or biochemical characteristics suggesting primary malignancy (Table 5.1) [1, 10, 11]. The size cut-off recommendations for surgery of an incidental adrenal nodule are based on reported malignancy rates, with lesions less than or equal to 4 cm with malignancy rates of approximately 2% or less,

4.1–6 cm with malignancy rates of approximately 6%, and greater than 6 cm with malignancy rates of approximately 25% [1, 10, 11]. The malignancy rate of lesions with a combination of indeterminate but suspicious characteristics is not well described, and therefore judgment is required when deciding on surgery and optimal surgical approach for patients with, for example, relatively small adrenal nodules with indeterminate imaging characteristics or those that demonstrate some degree of growth on serial imaging [1, 10, 11]. The decision to approach these lesions using a MIAS approach should be patient and surgeon specific [4, 10]. Recent studies have shown that the median average annual volume for surgeons performing adrenalectomy is 1 case [4, 10, 15, 16]. These same studies demonstrate improved outcomes when adrenalectomies are performed by high-volume surgeons (defined as 4–6 adrenalectomies annually) [4, 10, 15, 16]. For surgeons experienced in both TLA and RA approaches, and assuming the patient is eligible for either approach based on tumor type and anatomic considerations, a recent network meta-analysis of phase II/III randomized clinical controlled trials of minimally invasive adrenalectomy suggests that posterior RA is the best choice for patients with adrenal masses candidate for MIAS, because posterior RA was superior to other MIAS approaches in safety, operative time, blood loss, length of stay, and incisional hernia rate [4]. However, recent results from the Collaborative Endocrine Surgery Quality Improvement Program (CESQIP, 2014–2018) revealed a greater rate of capsular disruption with the posterior RA than the TLA (12.6% vs 7.6%, $p = 0.02$) and this was confirmed as an independent factor for capsular disruption in the multivariate analysis [17]. Therefore, the details of considerations provided in previous chapters help guide to determine the best operative approach. Tumor size affects the selection for MIAS approach, because larger tumors (≥6 cm) are challenging to oncologically resect through RA, due to small working space compared with the TLA [4, 10]. However, we must highlight that RA for small- to medium-sized tumors

(<6 cm) and confined to adrenal gland allows for minimal need to manipulate or grasp the adrenal gland or the tumor, minimizing the risk of capsular disruption, with the proven benefits for this approach [4, 10]. Patients who have had previous transabdominal operations may benefit from posterior RA to avoid potential adhesive disease [4, 10]. In addition, patient body habitus is also an important factor to consider, because morbidly obese patients with abundant intra-abdominal and retroperitoneal fat will demonstrate compression of the retroperitoneal space from their intra-abdominal organs secondary when in the prone position [4, 10]. Furthermore, such patients may have such a large distance between their abdominal skin and the retroperitoneal space, thus posterior RA permits effective access [4, 10].

No matter the approach, it is essential to respect oncologic principles in any lesion suspicious for malignancy. The tumor must be removed completely and intact [1, 10, 11]. Thus, the MIAS approach is considered preferable for lesions with atypical imaging features potentially representing an atypical benign lesion, for example, intermediate size, lack of intratumor fat, and growth on serial imaging [1, 10, 11]. In patients with clear evidence of primary ACC (adrenal tumor not suspected of representing a metastasis with necrosis, irregular borders, local invasion, or regional nodal involvement), the conventional open adrenalectomy is recommended to avoid capsular disruption, fragmentation, and improve oncologic outcomes [1, 10, 11].

5.4 Minimally Invasive Adrenal Surgery for Metastatic Disease

The adrenal gland is a common site of metastases from a multitude of primary sites due to the presence of multiple pathways of blood supply [14, 18]. Isolated metastases to the adrenal gland most commonly originate from the lung; however, other common sites of primary malignancy include melanoma, kidney, colon, breast, and lymphoma [19, 20]. Adrenalectomy in highly selected patients with isolated or oligometastatic disease from primary sites including the lung, melanoma, and kidney can result in prolonged survival duration and improved survival compared with similar patients who do not undergo adrenalectomy [10, 14, 18–20].

Metastasis to the adrenal gland should be considered in patients with an adrenal mass and a history of malignancy that tends to spread to the adrenal [1, 19, 20]. The patient should undergo evaluation for extra-adrenal disease. The evaluation required will vary by primary tumor type but may include whole body positron emission tomography (PET), dedicated chest CT, and/or MRI of the brain [1, 19, 20]. The decision to proceed with adrenalectomy for metastatic cancer is based on natural history of the underlying disease, tumor biology, presence of extra-adrenal disease, patient performance status, and availability of alternative therapeutic options [1, 10, 19, 20]. Adrenal biopsy has high sensitivity (92%), specificity (94%), and negative predictive value (100%) for distinguishing benign from metastatic adrenal tumors [21]. However, not every adrenal mass suspicious for adrenal metastasis requires biopsy. Newly identified or rapidly enlarging adrenal tumors unidentified on prior imaging in a patient with a history of a known malignancy with propensity to metastasize to the adrenal glands (e.g., lung, melanoma, renal cell carcinoma), are highly likely to represent adrenal metastasis [10, 21]. In such patients, and in the absence of an alternative systemic treatment or following induction systemic therapy, endocrine surgeons should proceed to surgical resection without preoperative biopsy [10, 21].

Whereas primary adrenal cancer is a locoregionally aggressive disease, adrenal metastasis is often confined within the adrenal capsule, offering more opportunities to obtain *en bloc* adrenalectomy [14, 19, 20]. In a multicenter European study of 317 patients who underwent MIAS and open adrenalectomy for solid tumor metastases, the investigators found that patients with renal cell carcinoma, metachronous lesions, and isolated adrenal metastases had more favorable outcomes than patients with non-small cell lung cancer (NSCLC), colorectal cancer, or synchronous metastases [20]. Patients with renal cell cancer who underwent adrenalectomy had a median survival of 84 months, NSCLC 26 months, and colorectal cancer 29 months [20]. Patients with metachronous adrenal metastases had a median survival of 30 months compared with 23 months for those with synchronous metastases [20]. In this study, 46% of adrenalectomies were performed using a MIAS approach, demonstrating the widespread application of this approach to patients with adrenal metastasis. Interestingly, their multivariate cox proportional hazards model, MIAS was associated with a survival advantage with a hazard ratio of 0.65 (95% confidence interval: 0.47–0.89, $p = 0.009$) [20]. MIAS has become the preferred operative approach for management of adrenal metastasis because it achieved the same level of results of tumor control and less trauma compared with open surgery [3, 14, 19, 20]. A retrospective review of 94 adrenalectomies for isolated adrenal metastases (63 open and 31 MIAS) found no difference in local recurrence, margin status, disease-free interval, or overall survival based on the surgical approach chosen [22]. Moreover, MIAS was associated with decreased blood loss (106 vs 749 cc, $p < 0.001$), operative time (175 vs 208 mins, $p = 5.04$), length of stay (2.8 vs 8 days, $p < 0.001$), and complication rate (4% vs 34%, $p < 0.01$) [22]. Ma X et al. evaluated in 75 patients with adrenal metastases an anatomical posterior retroperitoneoscopic adrenalectomy (PRA) [14]. The most common primary tumor was renal cell carcinoma ($n = 26$), followed by NSCLC ($n = 23$), and hepatocellular carcinoma ($n = 12$). A total of 76 successful PRAs were performed, with a median operation time of 53 (range, 40–250) min and median estimated blood loss of 25 (range, 10–700) ml. The local recurrence rate was 5.3%, and the median survival was 24 months. These data were comparable with or even better than other approaches in previous reported studies. The independent prognostic factors of survival were body mass index (BMI, $p < 0.001$), tumor type ($p < 0.001$), tumor size ($\geq$4 cm vs. <4 cm, $p = 0.017$), and margin status (negative vs positive, $p = 0.011$). Authors concluded that anatomical PRA could represent a safe and effective approach for the management of adrenal metastasis in selected patients [14]. However, MIAS, particularly the RA approach, may limit the ability to evaluate and treat other intra-abdominal sites of metastasis and may therefore be relatively contraindicated in patients with known or suspected extra-adrenal but intra-abdominal sites of oligometastasis for which concomitant surgery would be desired [10, 19, 20]. Therefore, when determining the operative approach to adrenal metastases, patient characteristics, tumor size, and radiographic evidence for local invasion should be considered.

5.5 Minimally Invasive Adrenal Surgery for Adrenocortical Carcinoma

Adrenocortical carcinoma (ACC) is a rare and aggressive malignancy that carries a poor prognosis [11]. Most patients present with locally advanced or metastatic disease not amenable to surgical resection. ACC has an estimated incidence of 0.5–2 new cases per million people per year and is commonly diagnosed during evaluation of symptoms related to hormone excess because approximately two-thirds of ACCs produce and release excess hormones [11, 19]. Complete surgical resection with negative margins is the only curative option for ACC. Thus, the operative approach chosen must have the highest likelihood of achieving this goal [11, 19].

Controversy continues to exist on the role of MIAS in surgical management of European Network for the Study of Adrenal Tumors (ENSAT) stage I (T $\leq$ 5 cm, N0, M0) and II (T > 5 cm, N0, M0) primary ACC. Proponents of the MIAS approach to ACC cite retrospective series that conclude that an MIAS approach is safe and can achieve similar oncologic outcomes for highly selected patients with relatively "small" tumors (<10 cm) without evidence of local invasion, provided oncologic principals are respected [10, 23]. In contrast, proponents of open adrenalectomy cite retrospective studies of referral populations of patients with ACC that have identified increased rates of peritoneal carcinomatosis, capsular disruption, positive margins, and recurrence, as well as poorer stage-specific survival, in patients undergoing MIAS compared with open resection of primary ACC [10, 23]. Some authors have reported poor oncologic results in terms of recurrence-free survival, overall survival, and uncommon type of recurrence (port site or peritoneal) after MIAS for ACC [24, 25]. Recently, in a systematic review, Autorino et al. analyzed nine studies, including 240 laparoscopic adrenalectomies and 557 open adrenalectomy cases [26]. At baseline, tumors treated with laparoscopy were significantly smaller in size, hospitalization time was in favor of laparoscopy, and there was no difference in the overall recurrence rate, time to recurrence, or cancer-specific mortality between the two groups [26]. However, development of peritoneal carcinomatosis was significantly higher for laparoscopic adrenalectomy. The authors concluded that open adrenalectomy should still be considered the standard surgical management of ACC, even if laparoscopic approaches can certainly play a role in this setting [26]. Two recent studies comparing open adrenalectomy and MIAS have been published [27, 28]. Wu et al. retrospectively evaluated data from patients with stage I and II ACC and tumor size less than 10 cm [28]. They were divided into open adrenalectomy ($n = 23$) and laparoscopic adrenalectomy ($n = 21$) groups. Patient baseline characteristics from the two groups were comparable, and mean tumor size was 68 mm in open adrenalectomy and 58 mm in laparoscopic adrenalectomy. Laparoscopic adrenalectomy was performed using the retroperitoneal approach in 12 cases, and the transperitoneal in 11 cases. One patient was converted to an open procedure because of tumor rupture. No differences were recorded in terms of perioperative variables, but shorter hospital stay favored a laparoscopic approach. The 5-year overall survival, and recurrence-free survival, rates for open adrenalectomy versus laparoscopic adrenalectomy were similar (43 versus 47%, and 36 versus 39%, respectively). However, when considering local and peritoneal recurrence (excluding distant

metastases) rates were 22% for open adrenalectomy and 42% for laparoscopic adrenalectomy ($p = 0.035$); moreover, time to local and peritoneal recurrence was less in the laparoscopic adrenalectomy than in the open adrenalectomy (40 versus 79 months respectively; $p = 0.048$). Authors concluded that open adrenalectomy should still be considered the standard operative management of ACC, because laparoscopic adrenalectomy may not provide patients with localized ACC with an equivalent oncologic outcome based on site and timing of initial tumor recurrence [28]. Similar data came from the Zeng et al. study [27]. They retrospectively analyzed the data of 42 patients, with stage I–III ACC, receiving open adrenalectomy ($n = 22$) or laparoscopic adrenalectomy ($n = 20$) as primary therapy. At baseline, the patients in the open adrenalectomy group had larger tumor size (10.1 versus 6.3 cm, $p < 0.001$) and a higher rate of stage III ACC (40.9 versus 20.0%). The perioperative data indicated patients might benefit more from laparoscopic adrenalectomy, because operative times, estimated blood losses, and hospital stay were lower in this group. Moreover, one patient in the open adrenalectomy group died of multiple organ failure caused by hemorrhagic shock 3 days after surgery. From an oncologic point of view, despite the fact that in the laparoscopic adrenalectomy group tumors were smaller and less advanced, patients undergoing open adrenalectomy benefited more than those undergoing laparoscopic adrenalectomy in short-term oncologic prognoses [23, 27]. The 2-year disease-free survival (DFS) of the open adrenalectomy group was 61.1 versus 21.4% for the laparoscopic adrenalectomy group. In terms of time to recurrence, the open adrenalectomy group showed longer mean DFS (44.8 months) than that of the laparoscopic adrenalectomy group (17.5 months). At statistical analysis, surgical approach was an independent risk factor for recurrence, which showed that the relative recurrence risk of the laparoscopic adrenalectomy group was 2.1-fold higher compared with the open adrenalectomy group. Five out of 13 patients with recurrence in open adrenalectomy versus 11 out of 11 in the laparoscopic adrenalectomy group, had local tumor bed recurrence [27].

On the other side, the role of lymph node dissection in treatment of ACC remains unclear; there is no consensus regarding the extent of lymph node dissection that should be routinely performed. Reported rates of lymph node removal in studies using large national databases are low (17–30%), but the rate of lymph node dissection is lower in adrenalectomies performed using an MIAS for ACC than in those performed open [29, 30]. Important missing data in these retrospective series is the proportion of patients who underwent lymph node removal of involved regional nodes for preoperatively or intraoperatively defined indications rather than routinely [10, 29, 30]. Furthermore, patients with primary ACC can present with formally resectable tumors, but with characteristics against immediate surgery, including a high risk for incomplete resection, early recurrence, or high risk of perioperative morbidity or mortality. Such patients should be considered to have borderline resectable ACC and be candidates for preoperative (neoadjuvant) systemic therapy [10, 31]. Early experience suggests such a combined approach with appropriately aggressive surgical resection, can result in good outcomes compared with patients treated with upfront open surgery [10, 31].

Finally, ACC is a soft tumor with consistency similar to friable adrenal cortex; capsular disruption and fragmentation are easy to induce, particularly during direct tumor manipulation that commonly occurs in attempted MIAS. Furthermore, ACC tends to invade through the tumor capsule with microscopic disease present at the gland surface; thus, minimizing direct contact with the tumor surface is essential to avoid violating the tumor capsule or causing disruption of disease at the surface of the gland [10]. The American Association of Clinical Endocrinologists/American Association of Endocrine Surgeons, the Society of American Gastrointestinal and Endoscopic Surgeons, as well as the European Network for the Study of Adrenal Tumors guidelines all agree that open adrenalectomy should be performed if ACC is suspected [11, 32, 33].

References

1. Araujo-Castro M, Guevara MI, Gutiérrez MC, Ramírez PP, Gimeno PG, Hanzu FA, et al. Practical guide on the initial evaluation, follow-up, and treatment of adrenal incidentalomas. Adrenal Diseases Group of the Spanish Society of Endocrinology and Nutrition. Endocrinol Diabetes Nutr (Engl Ed). 2020;67(6):408–19.
2. Sood A, Majumder K, Kachroo N, Sammon JD, Abdollah F, Schmid M, et al. Adverse event rates, timing of complications, and the impact of specialty on outcomes following adrenal surgery: an analysis of 30-day outcome data from the American College of Surgeons National Surgical Quality Improvement Program (ACS-NSQIP). Urology. 2016;90:62–8.
3. Staubitz JI, Clerici T, Riss P, Watzka F, Bergenfelz A, Bareck E, et al. EUROCRINE®: adrenal surgery 2015-2019- surprising initial results. Chirurg. 2021;92(5):448–63.
4. Alberici L, Ingaldi C, Ricci C, Selva S, Di Dalmazi G, Vicennati V, et al. Minimally invasive adrenalectomy: a comprehensive systematic review and network meta-analysis of phase II/III randomized clinical controlled trials. Langenbeck's Arch Surg. 2022;407(1):285–96.
5. Gavriilidis P, Camenzuli C, Paspala A, Di Marco AN, Palazzo FF. Posterior retroperitoneoscopic versus laparoscopic Transperitoneal adrenalectomy: a systematic review by an updated meta-analysis. World J Surg. 2021;45(1):168–79.
6. Constantinides VA, Christakis I, Touska P, Palazzo FF. Systematic review and meta-analysis of retroperitoneoscopic versus laparoscopic adrenalectomy. Br J Surg. 2012;99(12):1639–48.
7. Cooper AB, Habra MA, Grubbs EG, Bednarski BK, Ying AK, Perrier ND, et al. Does laparoscopic adrenalectomy jeopardize oncologic outcomes for patients with adrenocortical carcinoma? Surg Endosc. 2013;27(11):4026–32.
8. Miller BS, Ammori JB, Gauger PG, Broome JT, Hammer GD, Doherty GM. Laparoscopic resection is inappropriate in patients with known or suspected adrenocortical carcinoma. World J Surg. 2010;34(6):1380–5.
9. Leboulleux S, Deandreis D, Al Ghuzlan A, Aupérin A, Goéré D, Dromain C, et al. Adrenocortical carcinoma: is the surgical approach a risk factor of peritoneal carcinomatosis? Eur J Endocrinol. 2010;162(6):1147–53.
10. Kiernan CM, Lee JE. Minimally invasive surgery for primary and metastatic adrenal malignancy. Surg Oncol Clin N Am. 2019;28(2):309–26.
11. Fassnacht M, Assie G, Baudin E, Eisenhofer G, de la Fouchardiere C, Haak HR, et al. Adrenocortical carcinomas and malignant phaeochromocytomas: ESMO-EURACAN clinical practice guidelines for diagnosis, treatment and follow-up. Ann Oncol. 2020;31(11):1476–90.
12. Margonis GA, Kim Y, Tran TB, Postlewait LM, Maithel SK, Wang TS, et al. Outcomes after resection

of cortisol-secreting adrenocortical carcinoma. Am J Surg. 2016;211(6):1106–13.

13. Lenert JT, Barnett CC, Kudelka AP, Sellin RV, Gagel RF, Prieto VG, et al. Evaluation and surgical resection of adrenal masses in patients with a history of extra-adrenal malignancy. Surgery. 2001;130(6):1060–7.

14. Ma X, Li H, Zhang X, Huang Q, Wang B, Shi T, et al. Modified anatomical retroperitoneoscopic adrenalectomy for adrenal metastatic tumor: technique and survival analysis. Surg Endosc. 2013;27(3):992–9.

15. Anderson KL, Thomas SM, Adam MA, Pontius LN, Stang MT, Scheri RP, et al. Each procedure matters: threshold for surgeon volume to minimize complications and decrease cost associated with adrenalectomy. Surgery. 2018;163(1):157–64.

16. Lindeman B, Hashimoto DA, Bababekov YJ, Stapleton SM, Chang DC, Hodin RA, et al. Fifteen years of adrenalectomies: impact of specialty training and operative volume. Surgery. 2018;163(1):150–6.

17. Marrero AP, Kazaure HS, Thomas SM, Stang MT, Scheri RP. Patient selection and outcomes of laparoscopic transabdominal versus posterior retroperitoneal adrenalectomy among surgeons in the collaborative endocrine surgery quality improvement program (CESQIP). Surgery. 2020;167(1):250–6.

18. Lubomski A, Falhammar H, Torpy DJ, Rushworth RL. The epidemiology of primary and secondary adrenal malignancies and associated adrenal insufficiency in hospitalised patients: an analysis of hospital admission data, NSW, Australia. BMC Endocr Disord. 2021;21(1):141.

19. Glenn JA, Kiernan CM, Yen TWF, Solorzano CC, Carr AA, Evans DB, et al. Management of suspected adrenal metastases at 2 academic medical centers. Am J Surg. 2016;211(4):664–70.

20. Moreno P, de la Quintana Basarrate A, Musholt TJ, Paunovic I, Puccini M, Vidal Ó, et al. Laparoscopy versus open adrenalectomy in patients with solid tumor metastases: results of a multicenter European study. Gland Surg. 2020;9(Suppl 2):S159–65.

21. Harisinghani MG, Maher MM, Hahn PF, Gervais DA, Jhaveri K, Varghese J, et al. Predictive value of benign percutaneous adrenal biopsies in oncology patients. Clin Radiol. 2002;57(10):898–901.

22. Strong VE, D'Angelica M, Tang L, Prete F, Gönen M, Coit D, et al. Laparoscopic adrenalectomy for isolated adrenal metastasis. Ann Surg Oncol. 2007;14(12):3392–400.

23. Fiori C, Checcucci E, Amparore D, Cattaneo G, Manfredi M, Porpiglia F. Adrenal tumours: open surgery versus minimally invasive surgery. Curr Opin Oncol. 2020;32(1):27–34.

24. Gonzalez RJ, Shapiro S, Sarlis N, Vassilopoulou-Sellin R, Perrier ND, Evans DB, et al. Laparoscopic resection of adrenal cortical carcinoma: a cautionary note. Surgery. 2005;138(6):1078–86.

25. Miller BS, Gauger PG, Hammer GD, Doherty GM. Resection of adrenocortical carcinoma is less complete and local recurrence occurs sooner and more often after laparoscopic adrenalectomy than after open adrenalectomy. Surgery. 2012;152(6):1150–7.

26. Autorino R, Bove P, De Sio M, Miano R, Micali S, Cindolo L, et al. Open versus laparoscopic adrenalectomy for adrenocortical carcinoma: a meta-analysis of surgical and oncological outcomes. Ann Surg Oncol. 2016;23(4):1195–202.

27. Zheng GY, Li HZ, Deng JH, Bin ZX, Wu XC. Open adrenalectomy versus laparoscopic adrenalectomy for adrenocortical carcinoma: a retrospective comparative study on short-term oncologic prognosis. Onco Targets Ther. 2018;11:1625–32.

28. Wu K, Liu Z, Liang J, Tang Y, Zou Z, Zhou C, et al. Laparoscopic versus open adrenalectomy for localized (stage 1/2) adrenocortical carcinoma: experience at a single, high-volumecenter. Surgery. 2018;164(6):1325–9.

29. Reibetanz J, Jurowich C, Erdogan I, Nies C, Rayes N, Dralle H, et al. Impact of lymphadenectomy on the oncologic outcome of patients with adrenocortical carcinoma. Ann Surg. 2012;255(2):363–9.

30. Huynh KT, Lee DY, Lau BJ, Flaherty DC, Lee JH, Goldfarb M. Impact of laparoscopic adrenalectomy on overall survival in patients with nonmetastatic adrenocortical carcinoma. J Am Coll Surg. 2016;223(3):485–92.

31. Bednarski BK, Habra MA, Phan A, Milton DR, Wood C, Vauthey N, et al. Borderline resectable adrenal cortical carcinoma: a potential role for preoperative chemotherapy. World J Surg. 2014;38(6):1318–27.

32. Zeiger MA, Thompson GB, Duh QY, Hamrahian AH, Angelos P, Elaraj D, et al. American Association of Clinical Endocrinologists and American Association of endocrine surgeons medical guidelines for the management of adrenal incidentalomas: executive summary of recommendations. Endocr Pract. 2009;15(5):450–3.

33. Stefanidis D, Goldfarb M, Kercher KW, Hope WW, Richardson W, Fanelli RD. SAGES guidelines for minimally invasive treatment of adrenal pathology. Surg Endosc. 2013;27(11):3960–80.

Anesthesia in Posterior Retroperitoneoscopic Approach

Paolo Feltracco, Stefania Barbieri, and Michele Carron

6.1 Introduction

The posterior retroperitoneoscopic approach has become an increasingly used technique for resection of adrenal masses and isolated metastases to the adrenal glands. This minimally invasive approach allows direct access to the gland and may prevent unexpected lesions to intra-abdominal organs.

Technically, posterior retroperitoneoscopic adrenalectomy (PRA) requires retroperitoneal CO_2 insufflation and needs a proper learning curve in order to work in the retroperitoneal space, which is a relatively restricted area compared with the "insufflated" intraperitoneal space, as in the case of transperitoneal laparoscopic adrenalectomy (TLAdr).

PRA can be performed in the lateral position or in the prone (jack-knife) position, according to institutional or surgeon's preference. Studies and metanalysis indicate that the retroperitoneoscopic approach is superior to laparoscopic surgery in terms of reduced morbidity, postoperative pain score, blood loss, complications rate, return to normal activity, and shorter hospital stay [1, 2].

Implications and concerns of anesthesia for adrenal surgery in the posterior retroperitoneoscopic approach arise from the underlying clinical conditions/morbidity of the patients, positioning required for surgery, and potential side effects of high CO_2 absorption. Implementing an appropriate anesthetic plan, along with careful positioning and taping are mandatory to prevent hormonal/hemodynamic decompensation and skin, nerve, or bone injury.

6.2 Preoperative Patient Evaluation

A complete medical history and anesthesia-directed physical examination should be performed for all patients who undergo PRA. In fact, this procedure is currently also performed in patients with a wide range of risks of cardiac and pulmonary perioperative adverse events and surgical complications [3].

Preoperative evaluation should be focused on those medical conditions that may be affected by a potentially long procedure, in an obliged "uncommon" position, and that may "per se" affect the physiologic response to changes associated with anesthetics, fluid shifts, high insufflation pressure, and CO_2 absorption.

Patient preparation for PRA is undistinguishable to preoperative preparation for conventional laparoscopic or "open" adrenalectomy. Preoperative monitoring and management of electrolytes, blood pressure, and blood pressure lability should be

P. Feltracco (✉) · S. Barbieri · M. Carron
Department of Medicine, Anesthesiology and Intensive Care, University of Padova, Padova, Italy
e-mail: paolo.feltracco@unipd.it;
stefania.barbieri@aopd.veneto.it;
michele.carron@unipd.it

© The Author(s), under exclusive license to Springer Nature Switzerland AG 2023
C. E. Costa Almeida (ed.), *Posterior Retroperitoneoscopic Adrenalectomy*,
https://doi.org/10.1007/978-3-031-19995-0_6

implemented, particularly in patients with functioning adrenal tumors; adherence to specific medications, e.g., steroids in patients with Cushing's syndrome, alfa-blockade, beta-blockade, volume loading in patients with pheochromocytoma, should also be verified.

Preoperative cardiac risk assessment aims to identify unstable or undiagnosed cardiac conditions, estimate the risk of major cardiac adverse events, and determine who may benefit from additional testing prior to surgery. All patients need a thorough cardiovascular evaluation. Specially in patients with pheochromocytoma, a preoperative echocardiography is fundamental to assess global systolic function, valve function, as well as to outline the severity of potential diastolic dysfunction. Catecholamine-induced cardiomyopathy (behaving as a form of myocardial stunning), and significant dilated cardiomyopathy with varying degrees of heart failure, especially developing in case of longstanding tumors, should also be evaluated, or ruled out, as they can significantly raise the overall perioperative risk. Preoperative echocardiographic findings of moderate to severe left ventricular hypertrophy can be associated with both cardiogenic (from severe systolic and diastolic dysfunction) and noncardiogenic pulmonary edema.

The assessment of functional capacity in metabolic equivalents (METs) is recommended for patients with an estimated elevated cardiac risk [4]. Patients who have a poor or unknown functional capacity (<4 METs) can be further risk stratified with pharmacologic stress testing; the results would possibly change operative plans, perioperative pharmacotherapy, perioperative cardiovascular monitoring, the anesthesia plan, or even indicate the need for coronary revascularization [5]. Patients with a functional capacity greater than 4 METs can proceed to surgery.

Deep cardiovascular assessment and investigations may be required in elderly patients, as the combination of an unrecognized impaired autonomic homeostasis, an exaggerated response to anesthetics delivered, and a moderate reduction in venous return induced by temporary compressions of inferior vena cava (IVC) may reduce the stroke volume and compromise an already failing

heart. In elderly patients, the inability to compensate for the reduced venous return may be also related to the increased afterload potentially arising from intraoperative catecholamine release and/or to the loss of response to catecholamines due to receptor downregulation [6].

Coronary artery disease and impairment of cardiac filling and relaxation due to an often hypertrophied and stiff heart, along with persistent tachycardia not only increase the risk of myocardial ischemia but also decrease cardiac muscle work; these effects can be catastrophic in those with severe heart disease. Therefore, patients at risk and the elderly should be screened preoperatively for both coronary artery disease and "subclinical" heart failure. Patients with cardiac limitations and low METs undergoing PRA, even if less susceptible to serious hemodynamic effects when compared with intraperitoneal insufflation, are, however, more prone to develop postoperative hypotension and consequent risk for renal and other organ hypoperfusion.

Preoperative evaluation of respiratory function becomes important because of potential intraoperative respiratory effects of patient positioning and prolonged absorption of CO_2. In the lateral position, the dependent hemidiaphragm will be pushed into the thorax and therefore mechanical positive ventilation would require higher pressure as compared with the supine position. The dependent lung will also receive better perfusion while the nondependent lung would preferentially receive better ventilation than the dependent lung. This phenomenon will increase physiologic dead space and may lead to hypoxemia, especially if the dependent lung is already affected by disease.

As far as the effects of the prone position in anesthetized and paralyzed patients undergoing elective surgery are concerned, various studies have reported that the changes in respiratory physiology are generally advantageous [7, 8]. Pelosi and coworkers [9] have demonstrated that the prone position does not seem to have any adverse effects on pulmonary function, even in anesthetized obese patients. They reported, in accordance with other authors observations [10] that modifications in lung volume, lung and chest wall mechanics, and oxygenation do not occur over time during general anesthesia in the prone position. By turning the patient prone, the abdomen moves relatively freely, regional ventilation may increase in the more expanded, nondependent lung regions, with additional positive effects on oxygenation likely caused also by an unloading of the abdominal viscera and reducing the pressure on the diaphragm.

However, patients with chronic and almost debilitating respiratory disease may not show the positive physiologic response observed in a relatively healthy population, as the mechanical properties (compliance and resistance) of the total respiratory system may impede the proper adaptations. With patients who have Chronic Obstructive Pulmonary Disease (COPD) careful attention is needed when obtaining clinical history and during the physical examination in order to evaluate baseline symptoms, functional capacity and rule out active COPD exacerbation or respiratory infection [11]. Recent pulmonary function testing (PFT) is warranted in patients with new or worsening shortness of breath, changes in cough and sputum, active wheezing, or respiratory distress, and oxygen saturation lower than baseline. Even though in the majority of COPD patients, a preoperative arterial blood gas analysis will not significantly change the anesthetic plan, in patients with known or suspected hypoxemia or hypercapnia it may be useful. However, the following differential changes during PRA must be evaluated.

Patients with unstable COPD and those with exacerbations should be optimally managed according to most recent clinical guidelines [11].

Asthmatic patients should also be carefully evaluated and investigated since the perianesthetic period can be associated with life-threatening bronchospasm and status asthmaticus, particularly during painful procedures before anesthesia, induction, endotracheal intubation, and airway irritation during positioning [12]. The grade or severity of asthma should be assessed a few weeks prior to elective surgery to allow sufficient time for medical optimization.

A detailed history of the disease, with particular attention to specific triggering factors, previ-ous exacerbations, perioperative adverse events, need for previous hospitalizations and mechanical ventilation, current pharmacotherapy, and type of asthma control should be explored. Evidence of recent respiratory tract infection or poor asthma control (wheezing or diminished/absent breath sounds indicative of ongoing expiratory airflow obstruction) warrants further evaluation before surgery.

Patients with restrictive pulmonary disease should be evaluated with a physical examination and recent PFT. Preoperative optimization of these individuals, most of them under maximal baseline therapy, often reveals challenges, and delaying surgery, waiting for further benefits, may be risky from an oncological point of view.

Preoperative smoking cessation is still under debate; preoperative short-term smoking cessation seems to prevent harm for chronic smokers; however, the benefits are still to be confirmed on a large scale. On the contrary, various studies have demonstrated that an intensive smoking cessation strategy has been associated with reduced pulmonary and wound-healing complications [13, 14].

Despite scarce evidence in the current literature, preoperative chest physical therapy and inspiratory muscle training may also reduce postoperative pulmonary complications in high-risk patients [15].

6.3 Anesthesia for PRA

The anesthetic plan, as in general, includes the evaluation for possible difficult airway management, the choice of drugs for induction and maintenance of anesthesia, the possible need for large bore veins, central vein accesses, invasive hemodynamic monitoring, and body temperature measurement devices. Invasive monitoring of blood pressure through an arterial catheter cannulation is highly recommended, especially in hemodynamically unstable patients, coronary artery disease or other myocardial dysfunction, pheochromocytoma, Cushing's syndrome, and expected long or bleeding surgical procedures.

An anesthesia team comfortable with managing all adrenal pathologies (e.g., Cushing, pheochromocytoma), and with the prone patient position should preferably be available in the operation room. The primary aim is to deliver an anesthetic plan which provides stable hemodynamics in the face of potential catecholamine surges (especially at laryngoscopy, retroperitoneal insufflation, surgical stimulation, and tumor handling) or in the presence of an underlying significant cardiomyopathy.

General anesthesia with neuromuscular blocking agents and endotracheal intubation is always performed, as it allows optimal ventilatory control independently of patient position, facilitates elimination of carbon dioxide and protects against aspiration. In most cases, propofol is used for induction of anesthesia. Etomidate, still used in various centers for induction of anesthesia, is controversial in adrenal disease since it can suppress the adrenal function for 24 to 48 hours; anesthesiologists must be aware of this potential side-effect and be ready with parenteral corticosteroids if hypotension arises during the perioperative period.

Various inhalation and intravenous anesthetics can be used for maintenance of general anesthesia for PRA, depending on both patient risk factors and anesthesiologist's preference. The use of nitrous oxide (N_2O) for maintenance is not recommended; N_2O can be associated with a modestly higher incidence of postoperative nausea and vomiting (PONV) than other inhalation anesthetic agents (e.g., sevoflurane, desflurane, isoflurane); it diffuses into air-containing closed spaces, leading over time, for example, to bowel distention and potentially interfering with respiratory mechanics.

A lung-protective intraoperative ventilatory strategy should be applied with a tidal volume of 6–8 mL/kg ideal body weight, a fraction of inspired oxygen (FiO_2) of 0.4–0.5, and with PEEP of 5–10 cm H_2O, at a respiratory rate of 8–10 breaths/min. These settings maintain end-tidal CO_2 ($ETCO_2$) at approximately 40 mmHg and oxygen saturation (SaO_2) >94%.

The increase of the respiratory rate, rather than the tidal volume, is the first attempt to increase minute ventilation and compensate for CO_2 absorption while avoiding barotrauma. Mild hypercapnia (i.e., $ETCO_2$ approximately 40 mmHg) should be tolerated to avoid barotrauma. For severe hypercarbia (i.e., $ETCO_2 > 60$ mmHg) despite hyperventilation, signs of subcutaneous emphysema (i.e., crepitus over the abdomen, chest, clavicles, and neck) should be ruled out; if severe hypercarbia persists, reduction in CO_2 insufflation pressure is to be discussed.

Restrictive fluid therapy is recommended unless indicated for the specific disease, bleeding, or other needs; avoidance of fluid excess improves outcome and prevents bowel edema and interstitial fluid accumulation. In the case of massive bleeding or cardiovascular impairment, recovery of hemodynamics can be challenging, as heart rate, arterial blood pressure, and central venous pressure are unreliable to guide fluid therapy, and dynamic indicators such as stroke volume or systolic pressure variation remain controversial in this setting.

Once general anesthesia has been induced and the patient adequately monitored and stabilized, the patient should be turned to the established surgical position. Careful attention should be paid after proning to padding the face and other patient's parts of the body at risk of position injuries. The upper extremities are at risk of peripheral nerve injuries in the prone position. Perfusion of the arms should be monitored with palpation of pulses, visual inspection, and a continuous pulse oximeter. Sequential compression devices are usually applied for deep venous thrombosis prophylaxis. In some institutions, a mirror is placed on the table to allow the anesthesiologist to see the position of the endotracheal tube.

Some hemodynamic changes are to be expected just after turning the patient to the lateral or the prone position. In the lateral decubitus position, a reduction in cardiac output and mean arterial pressure can be observed. Mechanisms of this phenomenon include: variable reduction in venous return and preload for the right ventricle, as the heart is at a hydrostatic level above the lower extremities; lack of reflex tachycardia to compensate for drop in cardiac output (dampened baroreflex due to general anesthesia); the rise in intrathoracic pressure (which further reduces venous return), as abdominal content is not pushed away from the thorax.

Prone positioning can result in variable effects on cardiovascular physiology. As with the lateral position, a decrease in cardiac output is also seen; this is due to reduction of venous return, cardiac preload, and stroke volume. Blood sequestration in dependent body parts seems to be the main mechanism; other factors include partial caval compression, chest wall compression, reduced left ventricular compliance because of increased intrathoracic pressure, and mechanical ventilation with high PEEP [16]. Compensatory sympathetic tachycardia and an increase in peripheral vascular resistance may prevent the decrease in arterial pressure. Normally, an anaesthetized ventilated prone patient will respond to a fluid challenge.

Besides the significant management challenges to the anesthesiologist occurring during removal of functional tumors (e.g., pheochromocytoma), complexity of anesthesia conduction in PRA is also related to other concerns, above all, the potential hemodynamic effects of high insufflation pressure in high-risk patients, the consequences of excessive CO_2 absorption, and the practice of prone positioning.

Even though there is still controversy on the use of high insufflation pressure, retroperitoneal insufflation of CO_2 has been shown to determine less hemodynamic serious effects than intraperitoneal carbon dioxide insufflation. Despite initial considerations that higher insufflation pressure would decrease venous return and cause hypotension due to compression of the IVC, current practice has shown that patients generally preserve normal cardiac filling pressure and do not have appreciable reduction in cardiac output. The high CO_2 insufflation pressure (> 20–25 mmHg) commonly applied to increase visualization in the retroperitoneal space has been demonstrated to only moderately affect the inferior caval venous return. Since the artificially created retroperitoneal cavity is much smaller than the abdominal cavity, the adjacent vena cava can sustain a gradual, however consider-

able, increase in local pressure, and in non-volume depleted individuals, the impairment of circulatory function results negligible.

Giebler et al. demonstrated that in humans, retroperitoneal or intraperitoneal carbon dioxide insufflation evokes fundamentally different cardiovascular changes [17, 18]. They measured the inferior-to-superior caval vein pressure gradient and found that this caval pressure gradient differs with retroperitoneal or intraperitoneal insufflation for similar insufflation pressure. In contrast to intraperitoneal insufflation, the gradient between intra-abdominal and intrathoracic caval vein pressure remained unchanged with retroperitoneal insufflation of carbon dioxide until 20 mmHg of pressure. Furthermore, they observed that with insufflation pressure greater than 15 mmHg, intraperitoneal but not retroperitoneal insufflation resulted in the impairment of cardiac filling. Only above 20 mmHg and with right-sided insufflation, a significant increase in gradient developed. They also found a non-prominent increase in gastric or esophageal pressure with retroperitoneal insufflation pressure even up to 24 mmHg, which assumes that a smaller amount of pressure is transmitted from the inflated retroperitoneal cavity to adjacent tissues and to the peritoneal cavity than with intraperitoneal inflation.

Studies of hemodynamic changes during intraperitoneal laparoscopy in patients with cardiopulmonary disease have reported an increase in mean arterial pressure, systemic vascular resistance, and central venous pressure, with decreases in cardiac output and stroke volume during peritoneal insufflation [19].

Currently, PRA is increasingly performed since the common perception is that the retroperitoneal laparoscopic approach is associated with less hemodynamic disturbances and more cardiovascular stability than the transperitoneal approach.

However, during PRA for specific diseases such as pheochromocytoma, intraoperative cardiovascular instability remains one of the major operative and anesthetic challenges. Vorselaars et al. investigated in a large multicenter cohort study the different intraoperative hemodynamic effects of a transperitoneal or retroperitoneal approach for pheochromocytoma removal [20]. Multivariate analysis of their study showed that despite comparable overall and cardiovascular morbidity between the two approaches, the retroperitoneal adrenalectomy group was noted to have a significantly greater number of patients with mean arterial pressure < 60 mmHg, systolic blood pressure > 200 mmHg, and pressure volatility requiring drug therapy. Besides the worse results observed with PRA, authors' comments and conclusion were, however, that the operative approach appeared to only have had limited influence on hemodynamic instability during unilateral laparoscopic adrenalectomy, while the important event, consistently associated with detrimental cardiovascular effects, seemed to be the manipulation of the tumor.

In centers that routinely perform PRA, insufflation pressure > 25–30 mmHg is frequently used, and this condition is very infrequently associated with clinically significant hemodynamic and/or respiratory intraoperative or postoperative consequences. High pressure of up to 30 mmHg can be used because of the diameter of the tumor and anatomy of the retroperitoneal space, yet it causes only a minor increase in intra-abdominal pressure. Performing surgery at high insufflation pressure has been reported to be safe; in fact, it allows a sufficient working space in the retroperitoneum, facilitates early clipping of the adrenal vein, and by compressing the small veins, it keeps the operative field dry. Furthermore, since with retroperitoneoscopy there is little stimulation of the peritoneum, the sympathetic response and the catecholamine release is likely less.

The current literature, however, provides limited evidence to support the routine use of high insufflation pressure. Although the suggested benefits of high pressure include improvements in stroke volume, cardiac output, and mean arterial pressure [17], potential disadvantages on the contrary may consist of hemodynamic impairment in patients with low cardiovascular reserve (pressure of 25–30 mmHg in some individuals often flattens the IVC completely), along with pulmonary, and acid–base metabolic effects [20–22].

Recently, Billmann et al. in a multicenter retrospective cohort investigated whether retroperitoneoscopy with high pressure ($\geq$ 25 mmHg) compared with lower pressure (< 25 mmHg) reduces operating time and complications [23]. After propensity score matching, they found that perioperative outcomes, especially perioperative complications (bleeding, length of hospital stay, mortality) and operative time did not significantly differ between the groups. Considering that in their series neither patient safety nor operative success were compromised when PRA was performed with insufflation pressure below 25 mmHg, and that the operative procedure had to be temporarily interrupted due to hypercapnia in 2.8% of cases in the >25 mmHg group and 0.9% of cases in the 20 mmHg group, authors call for a careful re-evaluation of the routine use of high insufflation pressure during PRA. In order to prevent significant CO_2 elevations, they suggest commencing PRA adopting a strategy based on a moderate pressure, starting with 20 mmHg or less, and with the subsequent option of increasing insufflation pressure to counter intraoperative bleeding or exposition difficulties.

Carbon dioxide insufflation during retroperitoneoscopic surgery may cause respiratory acidosis and the diffusion of carbon dioxide into the body depends on the site of insufflation. According to many authors, the retroperitoneal space offers less of a barrier to carbon dioxide diffusion than the peritoneum [23, 24]. Streich et al. demonstrated that not only does retroperitoneal carbon dioxide insufflation cause more carbon dioxide absorption than peritoneal insufflation, but also absorption of carbon dioxide persists after the end of surgery [25]. In their experience, carbon dioxide absorption accounted for 40–60% of the basal value, with a tendency to increase steadily throughout the period of insufflation. In addition, at the end of exsufflation, carbon dioxide production returned to its basal value only in patients undergoing peritoneal laparoscopy, suggesting a persistence of carbon dioxide only after retroperitoneoscopy. Another study, on the contrary, after comparing patients undergoing PRA with patients undergoing open posterior adrenalectomy, found no difference in arterial carbon dioxide pressure, end-tidal CO_2, or arterial pH between groups; in this study the alveolar-arterial CO_2 gradient, however, indicated that absorption of CO_2 was higher during PRA [26]. In current practice, high CO_2 insufflation pressure in the retroperitoneum does result in demonstrable intraoperative hypercapnia mainly if operative time is unusually long and intraoperative ventilation becomes difficult because of the severe underlying disease of the patient or significant obesity. The reasons for the easier absorption of CO_2 include the high vascularization of retroperitoneal space and the high content of areolar tissue.

Despite the frequent carbon dioxide absorption/retention, and regardless of large interindividual variations, in patients undergoing retroperitoneoscopy, severe hypercapnic acidosis is infrequently a big concern as it can be prevented (even if not completely normalized) with proper adjustments of mode of ventilation. However, in order to adjust a high alveolo-arterial carbon dioxide difference, some individuals may require intraoperative ventilation with large tidal volumes and high respiratory rate, which become potentially dangerous, in particular with lung disease or prolonged use. Prolonged operating times are often associated with a greater predisposition to respiratory acidosis; therefore, especially during the learning curve, the selection of the procedure with a shorter operating time is recommended.

Surgery in the prone position is another important issue, as most anesthesiologists either remain relatively unfamiliar or become anxious with prone positioning. Although retroperitoneoscopic adrenalectomy in the prone position is considered the best approach for benign adrenal tumors because it provides the easiest access to the adrenal gland, it is not devoid of risks and complications.

Usually, anesthesiologists are not concerned with ventilating the patient in the prone position; as previously reported, mechanical ventilation has been revealed to be generally safe and the changes in respiratory mechanics are often advantageous [8]. However, in patients with respiratory dysfunction, or in obese individuals,

and in the elderly, the loss of elasticity of the airways and increased chest wall stiffness may potentiate the increase in airway resistance. The high resistance of pulmonary parenchyma and the low compliance of the respiratory system may make the adjustment of ventilatory setting, necessary to compensate for important hypercarbia, particularly difficult. When lung ventilation is increased, high ventilatory pressure in these "susceptible" patients may compromise venous return to the heart and result in hypotension, especially with the use of positive end-expiratory pressure.

Furthermore, in the case of inadvertent intraoperative hypoventilation or diaphragm displacement, lung collapse takes longer to resolve; this event, along with a tendency for poor coughing force, may lead to an increased risk of postoperative hypoxia and respiratory failure.

One of the major concerns for the anesthesiologist is the occurrence of severe complications associated with the prone position, namely, in particular, an accidental extubation and an unexpected cardiac arrest.

Even if anesthesiologists are trained to anticipate or plan for the worst-case scenario, accidental extubation in the prone position remains a very risky complication. Prevention of this serious event is based on the use of a reinforced and properly secured tracheal tube, whose patency, security, and correct position are to be checked and confirmed immediately before and after turning the patient. If for various reasons the tube become dislodged, a skilled anesthesiologist may attempt to reintubate the trachea with the use of a fiberoptic bronchoscope, otherwise the patient can be turned supine and subsequently reintubated without delay. Placement of a laryngeal mask in the prone position has also been done, providing a temporary patent airway until supination. The laryngeal mask has also been used as a conduit for the passage of a fiberoptic scope and successful tracheal intubation in the prone position. Another problem with this position is the risk of difficult removal of bronchial secretions in patients with chronic lung disease; cleaning of the tube by suction may be incomplete in the case of inspissated sputum plugs.

Cardiac arrest in the prone patient has occurred and been reported, and its management has been shown to be extremely challenging. The best way to treat this life-threatening adverse event is, whenever possible, to return the patient to the supine position, where the conventional maneuvers become more practical and advantageous. If for whatever reason immediate supination is not possible or it takes longer, chest compressions may be delivered with the hands on the central upper back, between the scapulae. Two-handed maneuvers can be also recommended; this technique provides better counter-pressure between the chest and the operating table and more effective compression of the thoracic cage. A "postcordial" thump delivered between the shoulder blades to treat pulseless ventricular tachycardia has also been reported [27]. Defibrillation in the prone position should be also attempted, with anterior and posterior paddles, or with paddles on left and right sides of the back; however, sufficient energy to the myocardium may not be delivered owing to anterior displacement of the heart and also increased transthoracic impedance with positive pressure ventilation [28]. Due to unforeseen intraoperative cardiac events, anterior and posterior self-adhesive pads should be placed before prone positioning in high-cardiac risk patients.

A reduction in cerebral blood flow is postulated in the prone position. Some of the mechanisms deemed responsible are raised intracranial pressure by increased intrathoracic pressure and by a reduction in cerebrovenous drainage from jugular veins, vessels distortion occurring from external pressure, e.g., from pillows or from flexion or extension of the neck, along with long rotated head position [29]. The potential reduction in cerebral blood flow should be considered, particularly in elderly patients or patients with vascular disease, where even modest reductions in cerebral blood flow would be significant. Careful attention to head and neck position (preserving the neutral position) should be paid during turning and while in the definitive prone position.

Other potential problems arising from positioning include injuries directly induced by pressure on the exposed area or indirectly by pressure to the vascular supply of the affected tissue. Injuries to the peripheral nervous system are not so infrequent (compression and stretching of ulnar nerve at the elbow, compression of common peroneal nerve or other superficial nerves); signs and symptoms of peripheral nerve injury (sensory or mixed motor/sensory) do not usually present early after surgery but rather in the following days [30, 31].

Ophthalmic complications ranging from corneal abrasions to important postoperative visual loss have been also reported with prone positioning [32]. Therefore, it is important that the eyes should be free from pressure and be checked regularly during surgery.

Specific complications of retroperitoneal laparoscopy with CO_2 insufflation at high pressure may include subcutaneous emphysema and air embolism. The insufflated CO_2 may proceed along the musculofascial planes up to the mediastinum, apical pleural space, and the neck. This emphysema, which manifests especially in case of long procedures, does not have a negative impact on the functional recovery of the patient and usually resolves within hours of the procedure.

Venous gas embolism may occur and is reported during retroperitoneoscopy. However, clinically significant emboli are very rare. Its incidence seems far less than the incidence reported during classical laparoscopic surgery [33, 34]. Since the retroperitoneal space contains less veins than the intraperitoneal space, the amount of gas under pressure reaching the systemic circulation due to possible severed or disrupted veins during surgery is therefore less. The typical signs of significant pulmonary emboli, such as unexplained hypotension, hypoxemia, abrupt reduction of $ETCO_2$ signs of right heart strain on ECG with a widened QRS complex, and arrhythmias, are extremely rare during PRA. In the unfortunate event that it occurs, supportive fluids and cardioactive medications, until cardiopulmonary resuscitation is achieved, may be necessary. Turning the bed and patient to the left side, and head-down position may allow the gas bubble to potentially remain in the right heart, thus delaying a massive bubble floating to the pulmonary artery (suggested but not demonstrated).

6.4 Postoperative Pain Management

Retroperitoneoscopic removal of adrenal mass results in less postoperative pain than the corresponding laparoscopic procedure (less peritoneal stretch and manipulation of abdominal tissues).

A multimodal approach to postoperative pain control including acetaminophen, nonsteroidal anti-inflammatory drugs, cyclooxygenase$_2$ (COX_2)-specific inhibitors, and opioid medication only as necessary, is generally implemented in many institutions. Rescue doses of morphine or pethidine may be administered for the first postoperative hours to reinforce analgesia provided prior to the end of the general anesthesia.

The authors' practice includes the routine infiltration of the incisions with local anesthetic at the time of wound closure, and postoperative administration of acetaminophen plus diclofenac in those where renal function is not at risk. Addition of tramadol, in continuous I.V. infusion, and exceptionally strong opioids, is implemented for moderate- to high-intensity pain or any breakthrough pain.

References

1. Perrier ND, Kennamer DL, Bao R, Jimenez C, Grubbs EG, Lee JE, et al. Posterior retroperitoneoscopic adrenalectomy: preferred technique for removal of benign tumors and isolated metastases. Ann Surg. 2008;248(4):666–74. https://doi.org/10.1097/SLA.0b013e31818a1d2a.
2. Nigri G, Rosman AS, Petrucciani N, Fancellu A, Pisano M, Zorcolo L, et al. Meta-analysis of trials comparing laparoscopic transperitoneal and retroperitoneal adrenalectomy. Surgery. 2013;153(1):111–9. https://doi.org/10.1016/j.surg.2012.05.042.
3. Raslau D, Bierle DM, Stephenson CR, Mikhail MA, Kebede EB, Mauck KF. Preoperative cardiac risk assessment. Mayo Clin Proc. 2020;95(5):1064–79. https://doi.org/10.1016/j.mayocp.2019.08.013.
4. Ganesh R, Kebede E, Mueller M, Gilman E, Mauck KF. Perioperative cardiac risk reduction in noncar-

diac surgery. Mayo Clin Proc. 2021;96(8):2260–76. https://doi.org/10.1016/j.mayocp.2021.03.014.
5. Duceppe E, Parlow J, MacDonald P, Lyons K, McMullen M, Srinathan S, et al. Canadian cardiovascular society guidelines on perioperative cardiac risk assessment and management for patients who undergo noncardiac surgery. Can J Cardiol. 2017;33(1):17–32. https://doi.org/10.1016/j.cjca.2016.09.008. Erratum in: Can J Cardiol. 2017; 33(12):1735
6. Wijeysundera DN, Pearse RM, Shulman MA, Abbott TEF, Torres E, Ambosta A, et al. Assessment of functional capacity before major non-cardiac surgery: an international, prospective cohort study. Lancet. 2018;391(10140):2631–40. https://doi.org/10.1016/S0140-6736(18)31131-0.
7. Edgcombe H, Carter K, Yarrow S. Anaesthesia in the prone position. Br J Anaesth. 2008;100(2):165–83. https://doi.org/10.1093/bja/aem380.
8. Pelosi P, Croci M, Calappi E, Cerisara M, Mulazzi D, Vicardi P, et al. The prone positioning during general anesthesia minimally affects respiratory mechanics while improving functional residual capacity and increasing oxygen tension. Anesth Analg. 1995;80(5):955–60. https://doi.org/10.1097/00000539-199505000-00017.
9. Pelosi P, Croci M, Calappi E, Mulazzi D, Cerisara M, Vercesi P, et al. Prone positioning improves pulmonary function in obese patients during general anesthesia. Anesth Analg. 1996;83(3):578–83. https://doi.org/10.1097/00000539-199609000-00025.
10. Nyrén S, Radell P, Lindahl SG, Mure M, Petersson J, Larsson SA, et al. Lung ventilation and perfusion in prone and supine postures with reference to anesthetized and mechanically ventilated healthy volunteers. Anesthesiology. 2010;112(3):682–7. https://doi.org/10.1097/ALN.0b013e3181cf40c8.
11. Costescu F, Slinger P. Preoperative pulmonary evaluation. Curr Anesthesiol Rep. 2018;8:52–8. https://doi.org/10.1007/s40140-018-0252-y.
12. Vogelmeier CF, Criner GJ, Martinez FJ, Anzueto A, Barnes PJ, Bourbeau J, et al. Global strategy for the diagnosis, management, and prevention of chronic obstructive lung disease 2017 report. GOLD executive summary. Am J Respir Crit Care Med. 2017;195(5):557–82. https://doi.org/10.1164/rccm.201701-0218PP.
13. Myers K, Hajek P, Hinds C, McRobbie H. Stopping smoking shortly before surgery and postoperative complications: a systematic review and meta-analysis. Arch Intern Med. 2011;171(11):983–9. https://doi.org/10.1001/archinternmed.2011.97.
14. Thomsen T, Tønnesen H, Møller AM. Effect of preoperative smoking cessation interventions on postoperative complications and smoking cessation. Br J Surg. 2009;96(5):451–61. https://doi.org/10.1002/bjs.6591.
15. Katsura M, Kuriyama A, Takeshima T, Fukuhara S, Furukawa TA. Preoperative inspiratory muscle training for postoperative pulmonary complications in adults undergoing cardiac and major abdominal surgery. Cochrane Database

Syst Rev. 2015;10:CD010356. https://doi.org/10.1002/14651858.CD010356.pub2.

16. Hatada T, Kusunoki M, Sakiyama T, Sakanoue Y, Yamamura T, Okutani R, et al. Hemodynamics in the prone jackknife position during surgery. Am J Surg. 1991;162(1):55–8. https://doi.org/10.1016/0002-9610(91)90202-o.

17. Giebler RM, Walz MK, Peitgen K, Scherer RU. Hemodynamic changes after retroperitoneal CO2 insufflation for posterior retroperitoneoscopic adrenalectomy. Anesth Analg. 1996;82(4):827–31. https://doi.org/10.1097/00000539-199604000-00026.

18. Giebler RM, Behrends M, Steffens T, Walz MK, Peitgen K, Peters J. Intraperitoneal and retroperitoneal carbon dioxide insufflation evoke different effects on caval vein pressure gradients in humans: evidence for the starling resistor concept of abdominal venous return. Anesthesiology. 2000;92(6):1568–80. https://doi.org/10.1097/00000542-200006000-00013.

19. Hein HA, Joshi GP, Ramsay MA, Fox LG, Gawey BJ, Hellman CL, et al. Hemodynamic changes during laparoscopic cholecystectomy in patients with severe cardiac disease. J Clin Anesth. 1997;9(4):261–5. https://doi.org/10.1016/s0952-8180(97)00001-9.

20. Vorselaars WMCM, Postma EL, Mirallie E, Thiery J, Lustgarten M, Pasternak JD, et al. Hemodynamic instability during surgery for pheochromocytoma: comparing the transperitoneal and retroperitoneal approach in a multicenter analysis of 341 patients. Surgery. 2018;163(1):176–82. https://doi.org/10.1016/j.surg.2017.05.029.

21. Kraut EJ, Anderson JT, Safwat A, Barbosa R, Wolfe BM. Impairment of cardiac performance by laparoscopy in patients receiving positive end-expiratory pressure. Arch Surg. 1999;134(1):76–80. https://doi.org/10.1001/archsurg.134.1.76.

22. Walz MK, Alesina PF, Wenger FA, Deligiannis A, Szuczik E, Petersenn S, et al. Posterior retroperitoneoscopic adrenalectomy—results of 560 procedures in 520 patients. Surgery. 2006;140(6):943–8; discussion 948-50. https://doi.org/10.1016/j.surg.2006.07.039.

23. Billmann F, Strobel O, Billeter A, Thomusch O, Keck T, Langan EA, et al. Insufflation pressure above 25 mm Hg confers no additional benefit over lower pressure insufflation during posterior retroperitoneoscopic adrenalectomy: a retrospective multi-Centre propensity score-matched analysis. Surg

Endosc. 2021;35(2):891–9. https://doi.org/10.1007/s00464-020-07463-1.

24. Wolf JS Jr, Monk TG, McDougall EM, McClennan BL, Clayman RV. The extraperitoneal approach and subcutaneous emphysema are associated with greater absorption of carbon dioxide during laparoscopic renal surgery. J Urol. 1995;154(3):959–63.

25. Streich B, Decailliot F, Perney C, Duvaldestin P. Increased carbon dioxide absorption during retroperitoneal laparoscopy. Br J Anaesth. 2003;91(6):793–6. https://doi.org/10.1093/bja/aeg270.

26. Brunt LM, Doherty GM, Norton JA, Soper NJ, Quasebarth MA, Moley JF. Laparoscopic adrenalectomy compared to open adrenalectomy for benign adrenal neoplasms. J Am Coll Surg. 1996;183(1):1–10.

27. Moore EW, Davies MW. A slap on the back. Anaesthesia. 1999;54(3):308. https://doi.org/10.1046/j.1365-2044.1999.0811z.x.

28. Walsh SJ, Bedi A. Successful defibrillation in the prone position. Br J Anaesth. 2002;89(5):799; author reply 799-800. https://doi.org/10.1093/bja/aef565.

29. Højlund J, Sandmand M, Sonne M, Mantoni T, Jørgensen HL, Belhage B, et al. Effect of head rotation on cerebral blood velocity in the prone position. Anesthesiol Res Pract. 2012;2012:647258. https://doi.org/10.1155/2012/647258.

30. Knight DJW, Mahajan RP. Patient positioning in anaesthesia. Contin Educ Anaesth Crit Care Pain. 2004;4:160–3.

31. Warner MA, Warner ME, Martin JT. Ulnar neuropathy. Incidence, outcome, and risk factors in sedated or anesthetized patients. Anesthesiology. 1994;81(6):1332–40.

32. Roth S. Perioperative visual loss: what do we know, what can we do? Br J Anaesth. 2009;103(Suppl 1(Suppl 1)):i31–40. https://doi.org/10.1093/bja/aep295.

33. Derouin M, Couture P, Boudreault D, Girard D, Gravel D. Detection of gas embolism by transesophageal echocardiography during laparoscopic cholecystectomy. Anesth Analg. 1996;82(1):119–24. https://doi.org/10.1097/00000539-199601000-00021.

34. Hong JY, Kim JY, Choi YD, Rha KH, Yoon SJ, Kil HK. Incidence of venous gas embolism during robotic-assisted laparoscopic radical prostatectomy is lower than that during radical retropubic prostatectomy. Br J Anaesth. 2010;105(6):777–81. https://doi.org/10.1093/bja/aeq247.

Technical Steps of Posterior Retroperitoneoscopic Adrenalectomy

Carlos Eduardo Costa Almeida

7.1 Introduction

Posterior retroperitoneoscopic adrenalectomy (PRA) is an easy-to-learn technique, with a short learning curve [1]. In a 2019 consensus paper from the European Society of Endocrine Surgeons (ESES), the learning curve for PRA was 20–40 procedures [2]. However, the learning curve is still a matter of debate since several factors have an impact on its length (see Chap. 11) [3]. The surgeon is one of those factors. If the surgeon already has laparoscopic skills from other procedures, the learning curve will be shorter [4]. Some authors report learning curves below 20 procedures [4–6]. Present in all these reports is the learning method. As with many other techniques, learning from an expert is advised [2, 3]; this is the best way to learn all the tips and tricks of this procedure.

This chapter aims to describe the technique in 10 standardized steps. Operation table setup, which instruments to use, and where to stand during surgery are important issues for making PRA easy and safe. Constant coordination among surgeon, assistant, and scrub nurse is of key importance. To keep the anesthesiologist permanently updated about the ongoing surgery and stressful steps of the procedure is also paramount for patient safety and surgery success (see Chap. 9).

The description of the technique includes 10 steps, which will help standardize the procedure in an easy-to-learn format:

1. Positioning the patient.
2. Placing the first trocars (balloon trocar and lateral trocar).
3. Creating the working space.
4. Placing the third trocar (medial trocar).
5. Finding upper pole of the kidney.
6. Finding the inferior vena cava (IVC).
7. Dissecting and ligating the adrenal vein.
8. Dissecting the entire gland.
9. Retrieving with an extraction bag.
10. Final check (hemostasis) and closure.

7.2 Surgical Instruments and Operation Table Setup

To perform PRA, you need common laparoscopic materials and instruments. It is a technique that all surgery departments can perform. A 30° camera and three trocars are used—one balloon trocar (12 mm), one 10 mm trocar, and one 5 mm trocar. The balloon trocar has a small balloon

Supplementary Information The online version contains supplementary material available at https://doi.org/10.1007/978-3-031-19995-0_7.

C. E. Costa Almeida (✉)
General Surgery, Portuguese Oncology Institute of Coimbra, Hospital CUF Coimbra, Coimbra, Portugal
e-mail: carloscostaalmeida@yahoo.com

around the tip which is insufflated with 20 ml air and allows the trocar to be fixed to the abdominal wall, leaving just the tip inside the retroperitoneum. The other two trocars are those commonly used in most laparoscopic surgeries.

PRA can be performed using only two instruments: a nontraumatic grasper and an energy device. We prefer to use LigaSure® 5 mm with a blunt tip. In this procedure, the curved tip of the LigaSure® Maryland can eventually help in dissecting the adrenal vein, though it is not crucial for a safe and effective procedure. Other surgeons may find it useful to use laparoscopic dissectors for adrenal vein dissection. You must know your preference and use the instruments with which you are comfortable. Finally, an extraction bag is mandatory for adrenal gland extraction.

For adrenal vein ligation, we only use LigaSure®, there is no need to use clips. During dissection, clips may fall causing a hemorrhage that may prove difficult to control. The energy device promotes a safe and effective ligation of both adrenal veins and adrenal arteries.

Good and correct patient positioning is crucial to perform PRA, which makes operation table setup of paramount importance (Fig. 7.1). One roll must be placed under the anterior iliac crests and another under the patient's thorax. This will allow for the abdominal viscera to fall away from

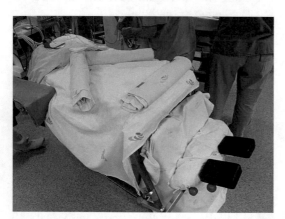

Fig. 7.1 Operation table setup. The rolls are placed to support the iliac crests and the thoracic wall. Attention should be given to the supports placed to support the bended knees

the retroperitoneum. The table must be set up to allow a nearly 90° hip flexure and to support the bended knees. We use adjustable supports attached to the operation table to help place it in line with the patient's body size.

7.3 Surgical Team

The surgical team is composed of the surgeon, the first assistant, and the scrub nurse. The surgeon and the first assistant stand on the same side of the gland to be removed; the scrub nurse stands on the opposite side. The screen must be in front of the surgeon, at his or her eye level. The surgeon will use both working ports, while the first assistant will manipulate the camera throughout the entire procedure.

7.4 Step-by-Step

Standardizing a procedure is very important in the learning phase. This standardized step-by-step approach is also useful at the beginning of the learning curve. However, changing one or more steps of the procedure may be necessary depending on the intraoperative findings. A good and expert surgeon must have the skills to adapt to each situation. The experience gained in different minimally invasive procedures is particularly important and helpful; what you learn in one procedure may be helpful in a different one. A surgeon who already has laparoscopic skills from other surgical procedures will be able to shorten the learning curve for PRA [4, 7].

7.4.1 Positioning the Patient

Only a good and correct patient positioning will make PRA safe and feasible. The patient is placed in a prone position. Arms are placed above and to the side of the head. Iliac crests and thorax are placed on rolls to make abdominal viscera fall away from the retroperitoneum; this is crucial for creating the working space. Thighs are placed in

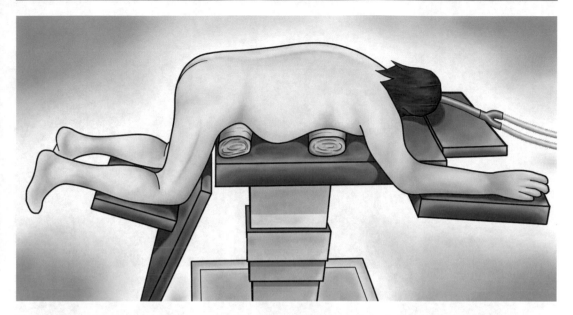

Fig. 7.2 Positioning the patient. Without correct positioning, PRA cannot be performed safely and efficiently

a near to 90° flexion position, with bent and supported knees (Fig. 7.2). Surgeons should take their time in this setup phase, as attention to detail will make the procedure easier.

7.4.2 Placing the First Trocars (Balloon Trocar and Lateral Trocar)

Trocar placement is a crucial step in all laparoscopic procedures. If wrongly placed, trocars will make surgery difficult, will cause pain in the surgeon's arms and back, will cause anxiety in the surgical team while struggling with the instruments, and will decrease patient safety. The balloon trocar (12 mm) is placed below the tip of the 12th rib (in all patients you can touch and feel the tip of the 12th rib). The 5-mm trocar is placed laterally and below the tip of the 11th rib. The third trocar (10 mm) will be placed in the midpoint between the spine and the balloon trocar (Fig. 7.3).

To place the balloon trocar, make a 1.5-cm skin incision with a no. 11 blade below the tip of the 12th rib. Go through the lumbar wall with Metzenbaum curved scissors and enter the retroperitoneum. Care must be taken not to injure the

subcostal nerve. Open the incision wide enough to place your finger inside the retroperitoneum. Touch the tip of the 11th rib with your finger. Under finger control, place the 5-mm trocar toward the adrenal gland (Fig. 7.4). Place the balloon trocar in the first incision, insufflate the balloon with 20 ml air, then pull and lock the trocar (Fig. 7.5). Insufflate the retroperitoneum through the balloon trocar up to 20–25 mmHg (we use 25 mmHg) [4, 8, 9].

7.4.3 Creating the Working Space

Before placing the third trocar, you must create a working space. Place the 30° camera in the balloon trocar, and work with the LigaSure® or a nontraumatic grasper. In the beginning, set the 30° upward. If the perirenal fascia is not open yet, open it with the instrument you are using. The objective is to pull down all the perirenal fat and create a wide working space. At this phase, the surgeon works with the camera and the instrument (Fig. 7.6). This step is completed when the surgeon sees the perirenal fat covering the kidney and the adrenal gland at the bottom of the image (Fig. 7.7).

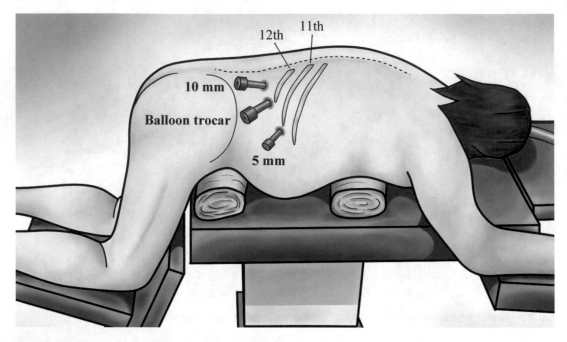

Fig. 7.3 Placing trocars. First incision will be below the tip of the 12th rib to enter the retroperitoneum

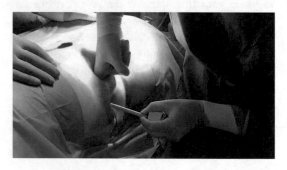

Fig. 7.4 Placing lateral 5 mm trocar. Through the first incision, place your index finger inside the retroperitoneum. Under finger control, place the trocar below the tip of the 11th rib toward the adrenal gland

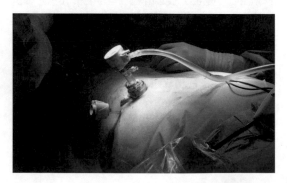

Fig. 7.5 Balloon trocar (12 mm) and 5 mm lateral trocar in place

7.4.4 Placing the Third Trocar (Medial Trocar)

Place the third trocar (10 mm) in the midpoint between the spine and the balloon trocar. It will be immediately lateral to the border of the spinae erector muscle. You must place it at an extremely acute angle toward the adrenal gland position. Control the entrance of the trocar with the camera.

7.4.5 Finding Upper Pole of the Kidney

This is the key point of the technique. A major difficulty for surgeons who are new to PRA is the lack of anatomical landmarks. In obese patients and in patients with Cushing's Syndrome you will only see fatty tissue. You must find a landmark to guide you throughout the remaining procedure. Finding this landmark—the upper pole of the kidney—can be challenging.

Move the camera to the medial trocar and set the 30° downward, pointing directly to the perirenal fat covering the kidney and adrenal gland.

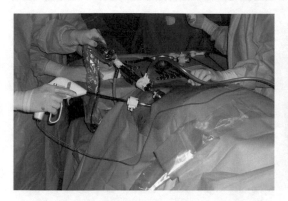

Fig. 7.6 The surgeon creates a good working space using a camera and instrument

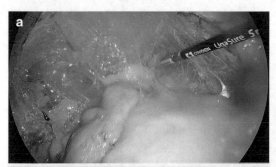

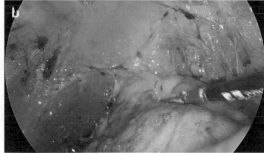

Fig. 7.7 Creating working space. (**a**) Pull down the perirenal fat. (**b**) Adrenal and kidney within the perirenal fat, after creating a good working space

Pull down the perirenal fat and the kidney within the fat. Start cutting through the perirenal fat from lateral to medial (Fig. 7.8). This will help avoid injuring the renal vessels. When the upper pole of the kidney is identified, pull it down, and cut the fat and areolar tissue between the kidney and the adrenal gland (Fig. 7.9). When this dissection goes medially, identify the inferior adrenal arteries and ligate them with the energy device.

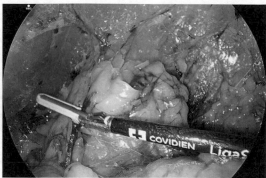

Fig. 7.8 Finding the upper pole of the kidney. Use the nontraumatic grasper to pull the perirenal fat. From lateral to medial, use the energy device to cut through the perirenal fat until you find the upper pole of the kidney

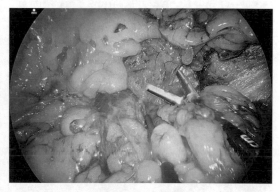

Fig. 7.9 Dissecting the adrenal gland from the upper pole of the kidney. Use the nontraumatic grasper to mobilize the kidney and cut the fat between the two structures with the energy device

Dissection during PRA has two directions: lateral to medial and bottom to top. The objective of the lateral to medial dissection is to find the upper pole of the kidney, separate the gland from the kidney, and leave the adrenal fixed to the diaphragm while avoiding the renal vessels. Since the gland is within the perirenal fat, you may not see it during the whole procedure.

7.4.6   Finding the Inferior Vena Cava (IVC)

In right-sided PRA, you will work close to the posterior wall of the IVC. After dissecting the gland from the upper pole of the kidney, you must identify the IVC medially and anterior to the gland. You must keep dissecting inferomedially to the gland, cutting all the fatty tissue, and using smooth blunt dissection until finding the "big blue," which identifies the IVC (Fig. 7.10). While conducting the referred dissection, "pinch and pull" the perirenal fat to be sure you are not grabbing the vein. When you have identified the IVC, use blunt dissection to separate the gland from the vein. This dissection goes "bottom to top" starting at the lower pole of the adrenal (Fig. 7.11). The blunt dissection should be done with smooth movements, close to the vein and along its posterior surface. Meanwhile, use the energy device to ligate medial adrenal arteries, which lie in a retrocaval position. This will help

dissect the gland from the IVC. Always use extra care when using energy close to the vein, ensuring that the venous wall is not pinched by the device.

7.4.7 Dissecting and Ligating the Adrenal Vein

The next crucial step of the procedure is to dissect and ligate the adrenal vein. Dissecting the adrenal vein may only be carried out with the energy device (LigaSure®), or with a laparoscopic dissector. The energy device may also be used to ligate and cut the adrenal vein; there is no need to use clips.

On the left-hand side, you will find the adrenal vein in the inferomedial aspect of the gland. After dissecting the gland from the upper pole of the kidney from lateral to medial, carefully ligate the inferior adrenal arteries. A long left adrenal vein draining into the phrenic vein and left renal vein will arise (Fig. 7.12). Grab the vein with the nontraumatic grasper. Use the LigaSure® to dissect, ligate, and cut the vein (Fig. 7.13). You can continue to grab the vein to help mobilize the gland during the remaining procedure.

On the right-hand side, finding and dissecting the short adrenal vein can be a difficult task. From the posterior anatomical perspective, the vein is found in front of the gland in a posteromedial position, between the posterior surface of the IVC and the anterior surface of the adre-

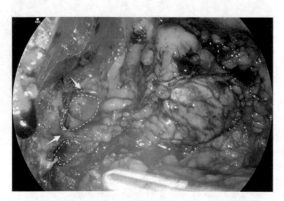

Fig. 7.10 Finding the IVC. The posterior surface of the IVC (dashed white lines) is found dissecting inferomedially to the adrenal. Medial adrenal arteries are crossing over the vein in a retrocaval position (white arrows)

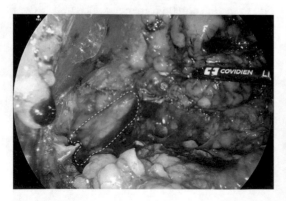

Fig. 7.11 Dissecting the gland from the IVC. Use blunt dissection to free the gland from the IVC (dashed white line). This dissection goes "bottom to top" starting at the lower pole of the adrenal

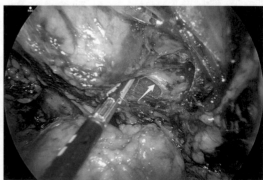

Fig. 7.12 Left adrenal vein. A long left adrenal vein (white arrow) in a patient with a 5-cm pheochromocytoma of the left adrenal gland

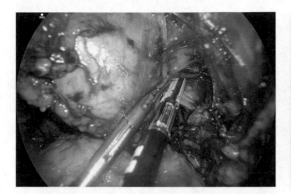

Fig. 7.13 Dissecting the left adrenal vein. Dissect, ligate, and cut the vein with the energy device. There is no need to use clips

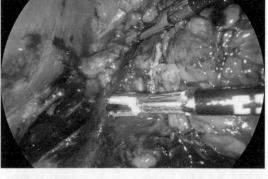

Fig. 7.15 Dissecting the right adrenal vein. The energy device can be used to dissect the right adrenal vein. Use smooth movements to avoid vascular injuries and bleeding

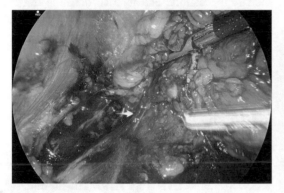

Fig. 7.14 Identifying the right adrenal vein. Gently lift the gland from the posterior surface of the IVC to find a small right adrenal vein (white arrow)

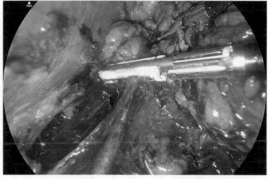

Fig. 7.16 Ligating and cutting the right adrenal vein with the energy device. There is no need to use clips

nal. The right adrenal vein usually drains directly into the IVC. However, be aware of possible anatomical variations (12.8%), especially a right adrenal vein draining into a posterior hepatic vein [10]. A good dissection is paramount to ligate the correct vein. Dissecting the right adrenal vein should be conducted with extreme care. Gently lift the gland with the grasper; with this movement, a small fold on the IVC is formed, identifying the location of the adrenal vein (Fig. 7.14). While keeping the gland lifted with the grasper, use the energy device or a laparoscopic dissector to smoothly dissect the adrenal vein (Fig. 7.15). Then, proceed to ligate and divide the vein with LigaSure® (Fig. 7.16).

7.4.8 Dissecting the Entire Gland

At this stage, the gland is separated from the kidney, the adrenal vein is already ligated, and on the right-hand side, the adrenal is almost completely separated from the IVC. The gland is only fixed by its superior adhesions. You must ligate the remaining medial adrenal arteries and the superior adrenal arteries, while dissecting the gland from the surrounding structures. Use the energy device to ligate the adrenal arteries and use blunt dissection to free the entire gland from the surrounding structures (Fig. 7.17).

On the left-hand side, you are close to the tail of the pancreas, the spleen, and the splenic vessels. Avoid opening the peritoneum.

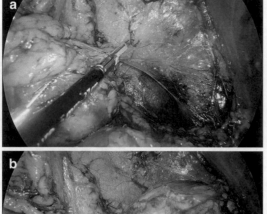

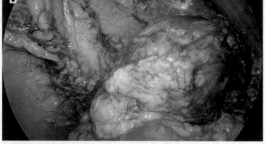

Fig. 7.17 Dissecting the entire gland from the surrounding structures. Use blunt dissection and ligate medial and superior adrenal arteries. (**a**) Use the energy device. (**b**) Left adrenal with a 5-cm pheochromocytoma fully mobilized and ready for extraction

On the right-hand side, pay attention until you have freed the gland from the IVC. This can be safely done with a combination of blunt dissection and energy. You are working very close to the bare area of the liver.

7.4.9 Retrieving with an Extraction Bag

After freeing the entire gland, you must retrieve it. Insert an extraction bag through the balloon

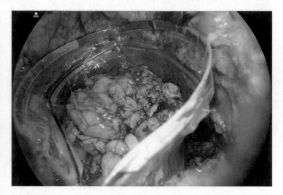

Fig. 7.18 Retrieving with an extraction bag

trocar. Place the gland inside the bag and close it. Deflate the balloon and remove both the trocar and the extraction bag with the gland inside. In big lesions, you may need to remove the gland in fragments. Introduce the balloon trocar once again and insufflate to 20–25 mmHg (Fig. 7.18).

7.4.10 Final Check (Hemostasis) and Closure

Wash the surgical field with saline solution and check for hemostasis (Fig. 7.19). The high pressure of the pneumoretroperitoneum tamponades bleeding of small vessels, and this can lead to a false sense of security. The pneumoretroperitoneum may be decreased to 5 mmHg and the surgeon may check for hemostasis. However, since the balloon trocar was temporally removed in the previous step, pressure has been zero for a while; if there is no blood accumulation when returning to retroperitoneum, hemostasis is good. A drain is not usually necessary. Close the aponeurosis and suture the skin as usual (Fig. 7.20).

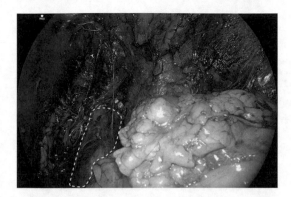

Fig. 7.19 Checking for hemostasis. The posterior surface of the IVC (dashed white line) is exposed after a right adrenal resection. There is no bleeding

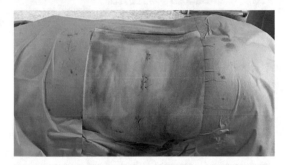

Fig. 7.20 End result. The patient cannot see the three incisions in the lumbar area. PRA has excellent cosmetic results

7.5 Tips and Tricks

PRA is a safe and feasible procedure. It is fast, effective, and has a low rate of complications. Experience and skills in laparoscopic surgery gained through conducting different procedures will help shorten the learning curve (see Chaps. 8 and 11). Knowing tips and tricks is paramount for performing PRA. Although working with an experienced surgeon is the best way of learning the technique [2, 11], the following list will help a surgeon to overtake some common difficulties he or she may find during this procedure.

- Place the trocars at an acute angle toward the adrenal. This is crucial for safe and comfortable gland dissection. In obese or male patients with a thick muscle wall, the correct place-
ment of the trocars toward the gland becomes even more important.
- In obese patients with Body Mass Index (BMI) >35, increasing pneumoretroperitoneum up to 30 mmHg can help to create a good working space [7]. Patients with BMI >45 are not good candidates for PRA [12].
- Increasing pneumoretroperitoneum pressure to 30 mmHg can also help tamponade bleeding of small vessels [13]. However, bleeding usually comes from small veins and arteries and is easily controlled by the 20–25 mmHg pressure and by the energy device [14–16]. We have never used clips for bleeding control, but they are a possibility if used with caution. Significant bleeding is a rarity. If that happens, applying compression with a gauze is the fastest and simplest way of controlling the bleeding [17]. See Chap. 9 for Management of Vascular Injuries.
- Finding the upper pole of the kidney is paramount to give the surgeon the anatomical landmark to go on safely with the procedure [4, 6]. This is the key point of PRA.
- Dissection must always be from "lateral to medial" and from "bottom to top" starting at the lower pole of the adrenal. On the right-hand side, dissection should be done in a clockwise movement from 3 to 9 h. On the left-hand side, dissection should be done in a counterclockwise movement from 9 to 3 h [13]. Respecting these dissection directions will help to avoid injury to the renal vessels.
- Retroperitoneal fatty tissue can be a problem while working in the retroperitoneum, especially in obese patients or patients suffering from Cushing's Syndrome. Removing the fatty tissue (e.g., by suctioning) around the upper pole of the kidney and the adrenal gland can help in exposing anatomical landmarks [14].
- The left adrenal gland has a different anatomical position than the right gland. Because the left adrenal falls in front of the upper part of the anterior surface of the left kidney, an extended mobilization of the kidney is mandatory to promote complete gland resection.

This will be easily achieved by applying pressure on the upper pole of the kidney with the nontraumatic grasper.

- The medial aspect of the right adrenal goes lower along the medial border of the kidney. This anatomical characteristic should be taken into consideration for complete gland resection. Inferomedial dissection will find the inferior adrenal arteries, which must be ligated with an energy device. You should pay attention to the IVC to avoid injury.
- When dissecting near the IVC, "pinch and pull" the fatty tissue to assure you are not grabbing the vein. If you feel no resistance when pulling, the IVC is free.
- Ligating the medial adrenal arteries which cross the vena cava in a retrocaval position may help to expose the IVC [13].
- From the posterior anatomical perspective, the right adrenal vein is behind the gland and in front of the IVC. It is usually a short vein that may be difficult to find and dissect. Gently lifting the right adrenal from the IVC will form a small fold on the posterior surface of the IVC, thus locating the right adrenal vein.
- Anatomical variations of the adrenal vein can be found on the right side (12.8%), they rarely occur on the left-hand side [10]. Typically, the right adrenal vein drains directly into the posterior surface of the IVC (87.5%). In 1.6% of patients, the right adrenal vein drains into a posterior hepatic vein, and in 6.3% it drains into the IVC just caudal to a hepatic vein. Other variations include two adrenal veins draining into the IVC (3.1%), or one adrenal vein draining into the IVC immediately cranial to the renal vein [10]. A good dissection and adrenal vein identification will avoid bleeding and inadvertent ligation of a hepatic vein.
- To keep grabbing the left adrenal vein with the nontraumatic grasper after ligation can help to mobilize the gland throughout the remaining procedure without capsule rupture. This tip is not valid for the short right adrenal vein.
- During Step 8 (Dissecting the Entire Gland), dissecting from "top to bottom" may sometimes help mobilize the entire gland.

- During PRA you may enter the peritoneal cavity from behind. However, because there is no compression of the retroperitoneum by the abdominal viscera, surgery can still be completed by using the posterior retroperitoneoscopic approach without taking any action [14].
- In rare situations, a fourth trocar can be placed below the line of the first trocars [14]. In a major vascular injury, it can be used to place a vascular clamp to control bleeding. In obese patients this trocar can be used for kidney retraction.

7.6 Video of Posterior Retroperitoneoscopic Adrenalectomy

All the 10 steps of PRA described above are demonstrated in a step-by-step video (Video 7.1).

7.7 Postoperative Care

At the end of procedure, the patient returns to the surgery ward. First oral intake occurs in the afternoon, and the patient stands up and walks. Acetaminophen is usually enough for postoperative pain control. Patient is discharged home the next day, only on painkillers (e.g., acetaminophen) as needed.

An exception exists for pheochromocytoma. Pheochromocytoma patients are usually preoperatively treated with α-adrenergic receptor blockers (e.g., phenoxybenzamine). The reason for using α-blockade is the reduction of both mortality and perioperative cardiovascular complications, including hemodynamic instability during surgery [18, 19]. However, according to Groeben et al., the indication for preoperative α-blockade is based on low-quality studies [18]. In 2020, these authors conducted a multicenter retrospective study of 1870 patients treated for pheochromocytoma or paraganglioma by minimally invasive surgery and compared those who received preoperative α-blockade (343) with those who did not (1527). Intraoperative hypertensive crises (arterial blood pressure peaks >250 mmHg) were identical in both groups ($p = 0.086$). Postoperative complication rate related to catecholamines-producing tumors (sustained hypotension, orthostatic dysregulation, sustained arrhythmia, cardiac decompensation, myocardial infarction, stroke, symptomatic hypertension, acute respiratory failure) was 5.9% with α-blockade and 0.9% without α-blockade ($p < 0.001$). The mortality rate was identical in both groups: 0.5% with blockade and 0.3% without blockade. Groeben et al. concluded that preoperative α-blockade increases preoperative orthostatic hypertension, does not decrease intraoperative hypertensive crises, does not reduce postoperative complications, and promotes sustained postoperative hypotension [18]. Although this study questions the utility of preoperative use of α-adrenergic receptor blockers in pheochromocytoma and paraganglioma (PPGL) patients, there are no criteria regarding which patients may or may not benefit from the α-blockade. Until more studies are available, preoperative α-blockade is the standard of care for all patients with hormonally functional PPGL, as advised by endocrine guidelines [19]. In that setting, we usually prefer that these patients stay in the Intensive Care Unit (ICU) for the first 24 h. The constant monitoring of heart rate and blood pressure of the patient in the ICU is crucial because of the possible hemodynamic complications, such as sustained hypotension during the immediate postoperative period. To avoid rebound hypoglycemia, glucose plasma levels should also be monitored in the postoperative period [19]. If everything goes uneventful, the patient can be discharged home after the second postoperative day. To confirm complete tumor removal, biochemical testing should be performed 2–4 weeks after surgery. A lifelong follow-up with annual biochemical testing is advised for PPGL patients [19].

7.8 Final Notes

Standardizing a procedure is the best way to learn it. The above description in 10 main steps aims at providing the reader with an easy-to-learn standardized sequence. However, surgeons must be aware that small changes to the surgical technique may be necessary to overtake unexpected difficulties during surgery. Having laparoscopic skills from other different procedures and having a solid background in surgical techniques can be of good value in a stressful situation.

The main difficulty for surgeons new to PRA is the lack of anatomical landmarks. The key point of the technique is finding the upper pole of the kidney. This step immediately gives the surgeon the anatomical landmark he or she needs to proceed with PRA safely and efficiently. Working with high pressures of pneumoretroperitoneum (20–25 mmHg) is also crucial to creating a wide working space. Additionally, incorrect patient positioning can make surgery impossible, so surgeons should take their time in the initial setup phase.

Prone position and high pneumoretroperitoneum pressures can be associated with stressful anesthetic situations (see Chap. 6). At the beginning of the learning curve, discuss the surgical technique with your anesthesiologist to make him or her comfortable with patient positioning and high pressures used in PRA.

The success of the surgery depends on the surgeon, the assistant, the anesthesiologist, and the scrub nurse. A preoperative briefing discussing the clinical case, the procedure about to be conducted, crucial technical steps, and possible pitfalls, will help increase the competence and confidence of the entire team.

References

1. Gimm O, Duh QY. Challenges of training in adrenal surgery. Gland Surg. 2019;8(Suppl 1):S3–9.
2. Mihai R, Donatini G, Vidal O, Brunaud L. Volume-outcome correlation in adrenal surgery—an ESES consensus statement. Langenbeck's Arch Surg. 2019;404(7):795–806.
3. Li R, Miller JA. Evaluating the learning curve for posterior retroperitoneoscopic adrenalectomy. Ann Laparosc Endosc Surg. 2017;2(12):169.
4. Costa Almeida CE, Caroço T, Silva MA, Baião JM, Costa A, Albano MN, et al. An update of posterior retroperitoneoscopic adrenalectomy—case series. Int J Surg Case Rep. 2020;71:120–5.
5. Bakkar S, Materazzi G, Fregoli L, Papini P, Miccoli P. Posterior retroperitonoscopic adrenalectomy; a back door access with an unusually rapid learning curve. Updat Surg. 2017;69(2):235–9.
6. Cabalag MS, Mann GB, Gorelik A, Miller JA. Posterior retroperitoneoscopic adrenalectomy:

outcomes and lessons learned from initial 50 cases. ANZ J Surg. 2015;85(6):478–82.

7. Dickson PV, Jimenez C, Chisholm GB, Kennamer DL, Ng C, Grubbs EG, et al. Posterior retroperitoneoscopic adrenalectomy: a contemporary American experience. J Am Coll Surg. 2011;212(4):659–65.

8. Costa Almeida CE, Caroço T, Silva MA, Albano MN, Louro JM, Carvalho LF, et al. Posterior retroperitoneoscopic adrenalectomy—Case series. Int J Surg Case Rep. 2018;51:174–7.

9. Costa Almeida CE, Silva M, Carvalho L, Costa Almeida CM. Adrenal giant cystic pheochromocytoma treated by posterior retroperitoneoscopic adrenalectomy. Int J Surg Case Rep. 2017;30:201–4.

10. Walz MK, Peitgen K, Walz MV, Hoermann R, Saller B, Giebler RM, et al. Posterior retroperitoneoscopic adrenalectomy: lessons learned within five years. World J Surg. 2001;25(6):728–34.

11. Perrier ND, Kennamer DL, Bao R, Jimenez C, Grubbs EG, Lee JE, et al. Posterior retroperitoneoscopic adrenalectomy: preferred technique for removal of benign tumors and isolated metastases. Ann Surg. 2008;248(4):666–74.

12. Walz MK, Alesina PF, Wenger FA, Deligiannis A, Szuczik E, Petersenn S, et al. Posterior retroperitoneoscopic adrenalectomy-results of 560 procedures in 520 patients. Surgery. 2006;140(6):943–8.

13. Alesina PF. Retroperitoneal adrenalectomy-learning curve, practical tips and tricks, what limits its wider uptake. Gland Surg. 2019;8(Suppl 1):S36–40.

14. Walz M. Posterior Retroperitoneoscopic Adrenalectomy. In: Dimitros L, van Heerden JA, editors. Adrenal glands diagnostic aspects and surgical therapy. Berlin. Heidelberg: Springer; 2005. p. 333–9.

15. Meraney AM, Samee AA-E, Gill IS. Vascular and bowel complications during retroperitoneal laparoscopic surgery. J Urol. 2002;168(5):1941–4.

16. Kumar M, Kumar R, Hemal AK, Gupta NP. Complications of retroperitoneoscopic surgery at one centre. BJU Int. 2001;87(7):607–12.

17. Asfour V, Smythe E, Attia R. Vascular injury at laparoscopy: a guide to management. J Obstet Gynaecol. 2018;38(5):598–606.

18. Groeben H, Walz MK, Nottebaum BJ, Alesina PF, Greenwald A, Schumann R, et al. International multicentre review of perioperative management and outcome for catecholamine-producing tumours. Br J Surg. 2020;107(2):e170–8.

19. Lenders JWM, Duh QY, Eisenhofer G, Gimenez-Roqueplo AP, Grebe SKG, Murad MH, et al. Pheochromocytoma and paraganglioma: an endocrine society clinical practice guideline. J Clin Endocrinol Metab. 2014;99(6):1915–42.

Intraoperative Complications

Francesca Torresan, Claudia Armellin,
and Maurizio Iacobone

8.1 Introduction

Minimally invasive adrenalectomy, either laparoscopic or retroperitoneoscopic, has largely replaced open surgery since it was first described in 1992. The initial enthusiasm was factually confirmed over the years; a retrospective comparative study between open ($n = 592$) and laparoscopic ($n = 1980$) adrenalectomy performed in the United States of America between 2005 and 2009 showed a 4.6-fold increased risk of serious complications, requiring Intensive Care Unit (ICU) care, and a 4.9-fold increased risk of mortality for laparotomy compared with laparoscopy, despite baseline comorbidities [1]. The excellent results of minimally invasive adrenalectomy have been published in many large series also in recent years, with the rate of intraoperative and postoperative complications reported in the different studies ranging from 0% to 15% for unilateral adrenalectomy, to over 23% for bilateral adrenalectomy [2–8]. However, despite the recognized safety and efficacy of minimally invasive adrenalectomy, the rate of intra- and postoperative complications is not negligible.

Nowadays, the most widely used minimally invasive adrenal procedures are the transperitoneal laparoscopic adrenalectomy (TLAdr), in the lateral position, and posterior retroperitoneoscopic adrenalectomy (PRA), in the prone position; nevertheless, also a lateral retroperitoneoscopic approach is performed in some centers, and robotic adrenalectomy is being improved [9].

The advantages of TLAdr compared to open surgery, such as less postoperative pain, shorter hospital stay, appealing cosmesis, and fewer intraoperative and postoperative complications, have made this operation the gold standard for adrenal lesions [10]. In a French retrospective study evaluating the complications observed in a series of 169 consecutive TLAdr (performed at the same center, for a variety of disorders), 12 patients (7.5%) had significant complications: three peritoneal hematomas (two of which required a re-laparotomy), one parietal hematoma, three intraoperative bleeding episodes without need for transfusion, one partial infarction of the spleen that regressed spontaneously, one pneumothorax, two deep venous thromboses, and one capsular effraction of the tumor, with an overall average length of hospital stay of 5.4 days (range 3–15 days); mortality was not reported [6].

However, many studies indicate that PRA is superior to laparoscopic adrenalectomy regarding operation time, pain score, blood loss, complications rate, and return to normal activity. The

F. Torresan · C. Armellin · M. Iacobone (✉)
Endocrine Surgery Unit, Department of Surgery,
Oncology and Gastroenterology, University of
Padova, Padova, Italy
e-mail: francesca.torresan@unipd.it;
maurizio.iacobone@unipd.it

posterior retroperitoneoscopic approach to the adrenal glands offers the benefits of the open posterior route and of minimally invasive technique, by a direct and minimal access to the area at the same time.

Between 1993 and 1994, the PRA technique was gradually implemented in different countries. Early descriptions were published from Turkey, the United States of America, Italy, and Germany [1, 7, 11]. Further studies demonstrated operative feasibility and—compared with the laparoscopic approach—shorter operative times and minor blood loss [12, 13]. In the largest series of PRA in the literature—560 procedures performed on 520 patients—Walz and colleagues reported a 2% conversion rate, a mean operating time of 67 minutes, and a very low complication rate (major complications in 1.3% of patients, minor complications in 14.4%) [8]. Intraoperative complications included pleural tears in four patients: these were managed by sealing the leak with pressure or by the placement of a pleural drain until the end of the surgical procedure, and in any case conversion to an open procedure was not required. Postoperative complications included one case of myocardial infarction, two cases of pneumonia, and one pneumothorax. Four patients developed postoperative hematomas, and one of them required a blood transfusion and reoperation. There was a significant rate of injury to the subcostal nerve (47 patients; 8.5%), which led to hypoesthesia and/or relaxation of the abdominal wall; however, these side effects were usually temporary [8].

Several retrospective studies have compared PRA and TLAdr [5–7, 14, 15]. Overall, these studies found a decrease in operating time and intraoperative blood loss with PRA and no difference in long-term outcomes. In two small randomized prospective trials comparing minimally invasive retroperitoneal and transperitoneal approaches, no differences in operating time, complications, or analgesic requirements were found, but both studies considered surgery by a lateral, not a posterior, retroperitoneoscopic approach [12, 15].

This chapter analyzes the complications of PRA, often in a comparison with the most performed TLAdr, using the available data in the literature.

8.2 Vascular Injury, Hemorrhage, and Cardiovascular Complications

The major potential complication of adrenal surgery is the arterial and venous bleeding: injuries to blood vessels represent the most common intraoperative complication of adrenalectomy, with a reported incidence up to 5.4% [16]. This high number of vascular injuries can be explained by the location of the adrenal gland and by its proximity to the main retroperitoneal vessels. In particular, on the right side, the adrenal vein is very short, and regularly enters the vena cava laterodorsally, so its exposure is the main risk for vein laceration, especially during the dissection of large tumors, which are inevitably associated with greater traction on the vein. A French series on the outcomes of laparoscopic adrenalectomy described four conversion cases (2%) in 204 right-sided operations after intraoperative injury to the inferior vena cava (IVC) [3]. These data are consistent with the results of a German series of 174 minimally invasive surgeries (144 laparoscopic and 30 retroperitoneoscopic), which also describes four cases of conversion for hemorrhage (2.3%), with no further discussion of the cause of the hemorrhage or whether they occurred during laparoscopic or retroperitoneoscopic surgery [14].

The posterior approach allows early transection of the transverse arteries originating from the aorta, thereby facilitating the dissection of the adrenal gland from the vena cava on the right side. Bleeding from venous vessels coming from suprarenal veins or IVC is usually well controlled by clips or compression. Importantly, anatomical variants of suprarenal veins on the right side, such as the common venous trunk between the adrenal vein and accessory posterior hepatic veins, may present difficulties in the dissection and can potentially cause harmful hemorrhagic events. However, given the restricted retroperitoneal space and the high CO_2 insufflation, the total blood loss is usually limited [17]. In fact, the high CO_2 insufflation pressures (> 20 mmHg) used to increase visualization in the retroperitoneum not only allow a sufficiently large working space, but, as an added benefit, compress small veins, minimizing bleeding and ensuring a dry field.

Although arterial vessel damage is less common during dissection, the renal artery or one of its terminal branches may be injured during both laparoscopy and retroperitoneoscopy. However, there is a lower reported risk of arterial injuries by PRA and the bleeding from small arterial vessels can be easily controlled by clips [17]. Most commonly, careless use of clips or vessel-sealing instruments may lead to unnoticed occlusion of the renal vessels and consequently to segmental infarction of the parenchyma, or, less often, to a complete loss of the ipsilateral kidney [3, 18].

Vascular injury can be also explained by incomplete exposure and accidental direct impact of laparoscopic instruments on the vessels wall or by their thermal damage. Intraoperative management of such lesions requires a high level of expertise in minimally invasive surgery and is the reason for conversions to laparotomy for endoscopically uncontrollable hemorrhage (see Chap. 9 for vascular injuries management). In the series of 560 retroperitoneoscopic adrenalectomies published by Walz and colleagues, no conversion due to vascular injury was observed, and other authors have reported similar results [8, 11, 19]. In a Dutch study involving 112 PRA performed in 105 patients, after operation one patient required re-exploration for persistent bleeding from the muscular part of a trocar insertion site, while minor complications, including flank hematoma, occurred in five patients [19].

The risk of air embolism is theoretically increased with the use of high insufflation pressures; this complication has been rarely reported [20, 21]. It may be caused by tears in large retroperitoneal vessels, mainly the IVC. In fact, normally, the high insufflation pressure during the retroperitoneoscopic approach keeps the vein compressed and does not permit significant bleeding or gas embolism; however, in some cases, a short period of accidental traction may keep it open permitting the embolism (Fig. 8.1). Moreover, while intraperitoneal filling pressures greater than 15 mmHg have been shown to decrease cardiac filling, retroperitoneal insuffla-

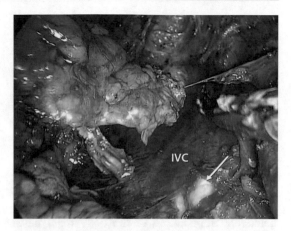

Fig. 8.1 Inferior vena cava (IVC) injury (white arrow) during right posterior retroperitone oscopic adrenalectomy

tion at high pressure increases stroke volume, cardiac output, and mean arterial pressure [22]. Furthermore, in reported extensive experience, no patient had iliac or femoral vein thrombosis or pulmonary embolism [8].

Although high CO_2 insufflation pressures in the retroperitoneum can result in demonstrable intraoperative hypercapnia, this condition has not been associated with clinically significant intraoperative or postoperative consequences. Interestingly, a recent study that compared patients undergoing PRA with patients undergoing open posterior adrenalectomy found no difference in arterial carbon dioxide pressure ($PaCO_2$), end-tidal CO_2, or arterial pH between groups, although the alveolar-arterial CO_2 gradient indicated that absorption of CO_2 was higher during PRA [23]. Hypercapnia appears to be potentially clinically significant only if surgery is unusually long, and the patient is difficult to ventilate at baseline because of obesity or underlying lung pathology.

8.3 Retroperitoneal Fatty Tissue

Adrenalectomy can present technical issues, especially in patients with a large amount of retroperitoneal fatty tissue, such as in those with hypercortisolism. These patients can benefit from an endoscopic approach that minimizes abdominal wall trauma. One of the major problems in these patients is the lack of an optimal endoscopic vision of the anatomical structures such as the main vessels. The resection or the suction of the fatty tissue around the upper pole of the kidney and the adrenal gland can facilitate the recognition of the main anatomical landmarks [17].

No specific studies examining the surgical outcomes related to large amounts of fat in the retroperitoneum have been carried out so far in the case of PRA, while some information is available about TLAdr. For example, Erbil and colleagues investigated the implications of the body mass index (BMI) and retroperitoneal fat area (RFA) in surgical outcomes of 51 consecutive patients who underwent TLAdr in a single center, finding out that in patients with high BMI, a high RFA was correlated to longer operating time and higher risk of complications, whereas low RFA was associated with significantly shorter operating time and decreased risk of complications; moreover, complications occurred in 50% of patients with both high BMI and high RFA, mainly because of technical difficulties and associated comorbidities [24].

8.4 Injuries of the Intestine

An accidental lesion of the bowel can occur both at the onset of laparoscopy (primary access) and during dissection. The incidence of bowel lesions after laparoscopic adrenalectomy is reported to be 0–1.3% [16]. Bowel lesions represent a serious complication, being responsible for 20% of deaths since approximately 50% of cases remain undiagnosed for more than 24 h [4]. The bowel may also be injured because of adhesiolysis, or during the dissection maneuvers, involving the duodenum on the right side and the colonic flexure on the left side. Retroperitoneoscopy in the prone position precludes bowel injury because the bowel remains outside the field of dissection. Therefore, it provides the most appropriate access for patients who have undergone previous abdominal operations, potentially presenting a high incidence of adhesions on the visceral side.

8.5 Injuries to Other Organs

All organs mobilized for proper exposure of the adrenal glands during TLAdr can be injured. Kidney and liver may suffer capsular lesions on the right side, whereas the spleen, pancreas tail, and kidney can be accidentally damaged on the left side. The real incidence of such complications is unclear, as most are small capsular lesions that are detected intraoperatively and remain without consequence. Complete mobilization of the pancreatic tail and spleen for left adrenalectomy has ample potential for serious intraoperative and postoperative complications. Rupture of the splenic capsule may be the reason for conversion or, if not recognized intraoperatively, may be responsible for postoperative hemorrhage. Injury to the pancreatic capsule, the incidence of which has been reported as high as 8.6% [19], can lead to pancreatic fistula or abscess formation. In a French study that analyzed the risk factors for complications of adrenalectomy in 462 patients, left adrenalectomy was the only risk factor for surgical complications [8]. In this series, 8 patients developed postoperative fluid retention in the upper abdomen, which required computed tomography-guided drainage in 6 cases. In all six patients, a postoperative pancreatic fistula was causative for the retention. In one case, surgical drainage was necessary in the further course of necrotizing pancreatitis. The kidney is rarely involved, with 3 segmental renal infarctions described in the same series after transection of upper renal polar arteries [8].

PRA offers undisputed advantages, as it does not require visualization and dissection of the liver on the right and pancreas and spleen on the left. Only the kidney is mobilized during retroperitoneoscopic surgery and may be injured. These capsular lesions can usually be managed intraoperatively without difficulty; renal hematomas, which may form postoperatively, usually do not require reoperation and can be treated conservatively.

8.6 Abdominal Wall Relaxation and Hypoesthesia

Relaxation and/or hypoesthesia of the abdominal wall are typical complications of the posterior retroperitoneoscopic approach [23]. Abdominal wall relaxation is characterized by a decreased muscle thickness of the affected area, without a gap in the continuity of the fascia, due to the injury of nerve structures, the subcostal nerves above all, during insertion of trocars and surgical maneuvers [24]. Longer operating times and larger wall incisions are often related to a higher risk of development of abdominal wall defect, and the higher density of nerve structures along the spinal cord makes PRA more at risk for this complication.

8.7 Pleural Lesions

Pleural lesions are also one of the complications of adrenalectomy, also for PRA. Recognition of this complication is usually straightforward because a pneumothorax or pneumomediastinum develops. The associated change in respiratory mechanics with increased ventilatory pressures and end-tidal pCO_2 as well as a drop in saturation do not go unnoticed by the anesthesiologist. Most lesions are not hemodynamically relevant and do not require therapy, suggesting radiological surveillance; otherwise, a chest drain, which is removed at the end of the procedure, can be inserted.

8.8 Misplacement of Trocars

During PRA, the peritoneum cavity can be accidentally opened; thus, in such cases, attention should be given to the abdominal organs that eventually become visible, such as the liver or the spleen. Nevertheless, the procedure can be con-

cluded by the retroperitoneoscopic approach since, in this case, an adequate working space is not precluded [17].

8.9 Rare Complications

Wound infections are also described in 1.2–1.4% of cases, with no significant difference in incidence between laparoscopic and retroperitoneoscopic surgery [5].

In addition to the surgical complications summarized above, general complications should also be mentioned. Pneumonia, pleural effusion, and pulmonary embolism, as well as cardiac complications (new-onset arrhythmias, myocardial infarction) and Addison's Syndrome, although with a lower incidence (<2%), have been described in all studies without exception [3, 8, 22]. It is worth mentioning the incidence of postoperative deep vein thrombosis and pulmonary embolism after laparoscopic surgery (up to 1.5% and 0.4%, respectively) compared with retroperitoneoscopic surgery, in which these complications were not observed [3, 5, 8, 22].

8.10 Risk Factors for Intraoperative Complications

Among different risk factors for the occurrence of complications during minimally invasive adrenalectomy, both patient's and tumor's characteristics affect surgical outcomes. Among the former, age and body mass, American Society of Anesthesiologists Class 3 or 4, and diabetes appear to be the most influent; among the latter, the tumor size, and a diagnosis of pheochromocytoma are the most important independent risk factors. Also, a mass larger than 12 cm in diameter and suspected malignancy are usually considered relative contraindications to minimally invasive adrenalectomy because of the higher risk of peri- and postoperative complications [4]. The risk of complications after bilateral adrenalectomy is markedly higher than in unilateral surgery (up to over 23% versus 0–15%) [2, 3, 7, 8]. Any procedural conversion (to hand-assisted or open surgery) is also associated to an increased rate of complications. Moreover, according to a study investigating the incidence of perioperative complications in TLAdr in high- and low-volume surgical departments, regardless of other risk factors, the whole number of complications, conversion rate, and non-surgery-related complications were statistically lower in the referral centers' groups (>30 adrenalectomies performed annually) than the non-referral centers [2]. Accordingly, both length of stay and charges seem to be significantly less for high-volume compared to low-volume centers [15]. Additionally, in a 2009 American study, 3144 adrenalectomies were analyzed to define the impact of surgeon volume and specialty (general surgeons versus urologists) on postoperative outcomes, concluding that patients with adrenal disease should be referred to surgeons based on adrenal volume and laparoscopic expertise irrespective of specialty practice [12].

In conclusion, both TLAdr and PRA should be preferably performed in high-volume specialist centers and by experienced surgeons. When available, robotic approach presents similar outcomes as laparoscopic adrenalectomy, especially for left adrenal lesions; however, clear indications on robotic adrenalectomy are still missing (see Chap. 12).

8.11 Laparoscopic Versus Retroperitoneoscopic Adrenalectomy

A summary of complications after adrenalectomy is shown in Table 8.1, comparing open, laparoscopic and retroperitoneoscopic approach.

TLAdr is considered a safe and standardized procedure, even for bigger tumors (>6 cm). The main advantage of the lateral transabdominal approach is that it allows gravity-facilitated exposure of the adrenal glands. However, based on the data presented, retroperitoneoscopic adrenalectomy appears to offer advantages due to extraperitoneal dissection, although these cannot be clearly demonstrated in a comparative study. A recent meta-analysis comparing laparoscopic (n = 1257), retroperitoneoscopic in the lateral position ($n = 471$), and retroperitoneoscopic in the prone position (n = 238) also failed to demonstrate a significant difference in postoperative complications. However, splenic injuries and intra-abdominal abscesses were observed only during laparoscopy or retroperitoneoscopy in the lateral position, whereas abdominal wall relaxation and hypoesthesia were documented only during retroperitoneoscopic surgery in the prone position [15]. Abdominal wall relaxation or hypoesthesia, while always transitory, was reported to have an incidence of 8.5% in a 2006 series [8]. In contrast, a prospective randomized study with 5 years of fol-

Table 8.1 Complications of adrenalectomy. Comparison between open, laparoscopic, and retroperitoneoscopic access methods

	Open adrenalectomy	Laparoscopic adrenalectomy	Retroperitoneoscopic adrenalectomy
Conversion due to vascular injury	–	2% [3, 23]	0% [8, 19]
Bowel lesions	Not investigated	Up to 1.3% [16]	Not described
Splenic injuries	Not investigated	1.2% [3] 1.7% [14]	0.7% [15] (in lateral position)
Pancreatic fistula	Not investigated	2.3% [3]	Not described
Abdominal wall complications	Incisional hernia up to 20% [25]	Trocar hernia up to 16% [13]	Trocar hernia 0.1% Hypoesthesia 8.5% [8]
Bleeding	Up to 5.7% [5]	1.5%	0.7% [8]
Blood transfusion	10.9% [23]	2% [23]	0.2% [8]
Pulmonary embolism	1.2% [1]	0.5% [1]	<1% [20, 21]
Pneumonia	Up to 5.7% [5]	2.4% [15]	1.7% [15]
Wound infections	4.6% [14]	1.2% [15]	1.4% [15]

low-up comparing 30 retroperitoneoscopic with 31 laparoscopic adrenalectomies found an incidence of postoperative trocar hernia of 16.1% after laparoscopy vs. 0% after retroperitoneoscopy [13].

Although conversion of laparoscopic surgery is not considered a complication, it favors peri- and postoperative complications. It has been calculated that conversion increases the risk of postoperative complications with an odds ratio of 6.2 [8]. Therefore, the experience of centers is important to reduce the rate of conversion, as demonstrated in an Italian study. In this study, the authors compared the rate of conversion of reference centers (>30 adrenalectomies per year) and other hospitals (<30 adrenalectomies per year) and observed a significant reduction in conversions from 6.0% to 1.6% in favor of the reference centers ($p = 0.003$) [2]. Therefore, the minimum volume regulation already implemented for other surgeries could lead to an improvement in the quality of adrenal surgery, because the appropriate experience can significantly reduce the risk of postoperative complications.

References

1. Eichhorn-Wharry LI, Talpos GB, Rubinfeld I. Laparoscopic versus open adrenalectomy: another look at outcome using the Clavien classification system. Surgery. 2012;152:1090–5.
2. Bergamini C, Martellucci J, Tozzi F, Valeri A. Complications in laparoscopic adrenalectomy: the value of experience. Surg Endosc. 2011;25(12):3845–51.
3. Gaujoux S, Bonnet S, Leconte M, Zohar S, Bertherat J, Bertagna X, et al. Risk factors for conversion and complications after unilateral laparoscopic adrenalectomy. Br J Surg. 2011;98(10):1392–9.
4. Hanssen WEJ, Kuhry E, Casseres YA, De Herder WW, Steyerberg EW, Bonjer HJ. Safety and efficacy of endoscopic retroperitoneal adrenalectomy. Br J Surg. 2006;93(6):715–9.
5. Hauch A, Al-Qurayshi Z, Kandil E. Factors associated with higher risk of complications after adrenal surgery. Ann Surg Oncol. 2015;22(1):103–10.
6. Henry JF, Defechereux T, Raffaelli M, Lubrano D, Gramatica L. Complications of laparoscopic adrenalectomy: results of 169 consecutive procedures. World J Surg. 2000;24(11):1342–6.
7. Kazaure HS, Roman SA, Sosa JA. Adrenalectomy in older Americans has increased morbidity and mortality: an analysis of 6,416 patients. Ann Surg Oncol. 2011;18(10):2714–21.
8. Walz MK, Alesina PF, Wenger FA, Deligiannis A, Szuczik E, Petersenn S, et al. Posterior retroperitoneoscopic adrenalectomy—results of 560 procedures in 520 patients. Surgery. 2006;140(6):943–50.
9. Kwak J, Lee KE. Minimally invasive adrenal surgery. Endocrinol Metab. 2020;35(4):774–83.
10. Smith CD, Weber CJ, Amerson JR. Laparoscopic adrenalectomy: new gold standard. World J Surg. 1999;23(4):389–96.
11. Dickson PV, Jimenez C, Chisholm GB, Kennamer DL, Ng C, Grubbs EG, et al. Posterior retroperitoneoscopic adrenalectomy: a contemporary American experience. J Am Coll Surg. 2011;212(4):659–65.
12. Park HS, Roman SA, Sosa JA. Outcomes from 3144 adrenalectomies in the United States: which matters more, surgeon volume or specialty? Arch Surg. 2009;144(11):1060–7.
13. Barczyński M, Konturek A, Nowak W. Randomized clinical trial of posterior retroperitoneoscopic adrenalectomy versus lateral transperitoneal laparoscopic adrenalectomy with a 5-year follow-up. Ann Surg. 2014;260(5):740–7.
14. Lachenmayer A, Cupisti K, Wolf A, Raffel A, Schott M, Willenberg HS, et al. Trends in adrenal surgery: institutional review of 528 consecutive adrenalectomies. Langenbeck's Arch Surg. 2012;397(7):1099–107.
15. Constantinides VA, Christakis I, Touska P, Palazzo FF. Systematic review and meta-analysis of retroperitoneoscopic versus laparoscopic adrenalectomy. Br J Surg. 2012;99(12):1639–48.
16. Strebel RT, Müntener M, Sulser T. Intraoperative complications of laparoscopic adrenalectomy. World J Urol. 2008;26(6):555–60.
17. Posterior WM, Adrenalectomy R. In: Dimitros L, van Heerden JA, editors. Adrenal glands diagnostic aspects and surgical therapy. Berlin. Heidelberg: Springer; 2005. p. 333–9.
18. Tessier DJ, Iglesias R, Chapman WC, Kercher K, Matthews BD, Gorden DL, et al. Previously unreported high-grade complications of adrenalectomy. Surg Endosc Other Interv Tech. 2009;23(1):97–102.
19. Schreinemakers JMJ, Kiela GJ, Valk GD, Vriens MR, Rinkes IHMB. Retroperitoneal endoscopic adrenalectomy is safe and effective. Br J Surg. 2010;97(11):1667–72.
20. Abraham MA, Josc R, Paul MJ. Seesawing end-tidal carbon dioxide: portent of critical carbon dioxide embolism in retroperitoneoscopy. BMJ Case Rep. 2018;2018:12–5.
21. Sollazzi L, Perilli V, Punzo G, Ciocchetti P, Raffaelli M, Bellantone RLC. Suspect carbon dioxide embolism during retroperitoneoscopic adrenalectomy. Eur Rev Med Pharmacol Sci. 2011;15(12):1478–82.
22. Chandler JG, Corson SL, Way LW. Three spectra of laparoscopic entry access injuries. J Am Coll Surg. 2001;192(4):478–90.
23. Bittner JG 4th, Gershuni VM, Matthews BD, Moley JF, Brunt LM. Risk factors affecting operative approach, conversion, and morbidity for adrenalectomy: a sin-

gle-institution series of 402 patients. Surg Endosc. 2013;27(7):2342–50.

24. Erbil Y, Barbaros U, Sari S, Agcaoglu O, Salmaslioglu A, Ozarmagan S. The effect of retroperitoneal fat mass on surgical outcomes in patients performing laparoscopic adrenalectomy: the effect of fat tissue in adrenalectomy. Surg Innov. 2010;17(2):114–9.

25. Seiler CM, Diener MK. Which abdominal incisions predispose for incisional hernias? Chirurg. 2010;81(3):186–91.

Management of Vascular Injuries (IVC)

9

Carlos Eduardo Costa Almeida

9.1 Introduction

Minimally invasive surgery has undergone revolutionary changes in the last decades, with more complex procedures being performed by means of different approaches. This revolution has been possible thanks to the existence of new surgical devices and better image capture devices. Complex and extended resections and reconstructions are now being performed safely and with good outcomes. Surgeons have increased their laparoscopic skills to such a high level that almost anything will be possible in a near future. From a diagnostic tool, laparoscopy has become a complex and sophisticated treatment method. As more and more studies have concluded regarding the safety, feasibility and successful outcomes of laparoscopic techniques, minimally invasive surgery has become the gold standard for the treatment of an increasingly large number of surgical diseases. Posterior retroperitoneoscopic adrenalectomy (PRA) is one of those innovative techniques. It is a product of the laparoscopic revolution, stemming from the need for being less aggressive and promoting faster recovery.

The consequence of this minimally invasive surgery revolution is the occurrence of more complex and severe complications than the ones seen when laparoscopy first started being used [1, 2]. Present-day surgeons need not only to have, but also explore and develop their skills so that they can deal with adversity laparoscopically. However, surgeons must not forget that the patients' well-being always comes first. Conversion to open surgery must not be seen as a failure but as an option to correctly treat a complex complication.

9.2 The Major Vascular Complication

Retroperitoneoscopic surgery (renal and adrenal) has several advantages over the laparoscopic approach. It has a low rate of complications, most of them minor [2, 3]. PRA has a lower complication rate than laparoscopic adrenalectomy. Additionally, PRA has less operation time, less postoperative pain, less blood loss, and faster recovery to normal activity [4].

Major vascular complications during minimally invasive procedures are rare but can be fatal. The global incidence of vascular injuries in minimally invasive surgery is 0.2/1000 procedures. These injuries are associated with a morbidity rate of 6–13% and mortality of 12–23% [5].

C. E. Costa Almeida (✉)
General Surgery, Portuguese Oncology Institute of Coimbra, Hospital CUF Coimbra, Coimbra, Portugal
e-mail:carloscostaalmeida@yahoo.com

Minimally invasive adrenalectomy (laparoscopic and retroperitoneoscopic) has an overall complication rate of 0–15% for unilateral surgery and up to 23% for bilateral [4]. In one of the largest published series on PRA, the complication rate goes up to 14.4% [3]. Even though the most common complications are vascular and visceral injuries during the transperitoneal laparoscopic approach (TLA), there are no data available on the rate of vascular complications during PRA [1]. In a 560 PRA analysis from Walz et al., no major vascular injury was reported [3]. As the retroperitoneoscopic approach (RA) is increasingly used, reports of complications will allow us to assess their frequency and severity [2]. Meraney et al. report a vascular complications rate of 1.7% during 404 retroperitoneoscopic procedures, including renal surgery and adrenal surgery [1]. These authors present a total of five vascular complications affecting renal veins and renal arteries during nephrectomies, and adrenal vein during adrenalectomy. They were able to laparoscopically control the bleeding with EndoGIA or vascular clips because all injured vessels could be ligated during the procedure. However, there may be an injury to a vessel which must be repaired and preserved. This not only increases difficulty but also demands vascular suture skills. In an analysis of 316 retroperitoneoscopic urologic procedures (renal and adrenal), Kumar et al. report seven major vascular complications. However, none of these complications (0%) occurred during adrenal surgery [2].

Vascular injuries during laparoscopic surgery can occur at entry (75%) or during dissection (25%) [2, 5]. Because the umbilicus is the preferred location for the Veress needle and first trocar placement in laparoscopy, bifurcation of aorta and the inferior vena cava (IVC) are the most common sites of injury at entry. Over 70% of injuries occur on the right-side iliac vessels, possibly because of trocar trajectory during placement, considering that the surgeon is standing on the patient's left side in many laparoscopic procedures [5]. In PRA, there is no risk for vascular injury at entry, since first trocar is placed with digital control and no Veress needle is used. Vascular injuries will only occur during dissection (blunt, sharp, or energy devices). During a PRA, major vascular complications may include injury to the IVC above the renal vessels, injury to the renal veins, and injury to the renal arteries. In all these scenarios, the surgeon must repair and preserve the vessel. Minor vascular bleeding can stop spontaneously due to the high pneumoretroperitoneum pressure [2, 4].

In a review of 31 cases of major vascular injuries during gynecologic laparoscopic surgery, all fatalities (22.6%) were due to venous damage on the right or left side [6]. This data supports the idea that it is easier to repair an artery than a vein. Arteries and veins are anatomically different. A major artery is composed of an endothelium, an internal elastic lamina, a thick layer of muscle and elastic fibers, an external elastic lamina, and an adventitia with vasa vasorum. In contrast, a major vein has a thin layer of muscle fibers, no elastic laminas, and the adventitia is the thickest layer. The vein has a thin wall compared to the large lumen. Additionally, the diameter of the arterial lumen is identical to the wall thickness [7]. Due to these anatomical characteristics, a vein ruptures easily during repair even if the surgeon's hand movement is smooth.

9.3 Surgical Team and Operation Room Staff Preparation

A retrospective analysis of 89 cases of retroperitoneal major vascular injuries (aorta and/or IVC) following blunt and penetrating trauma treated in a Level 1 Trauma Center concluded that factors for reducing mortality include spending less time from the admission to the operation stage, aggressive resuscitation method, as well as having human and material resources ready [8].

In elective surgery, the patient is already in the operation room, but it is crucial that the surgical team, anesthesiologist, scrub nurse as well as the remaining operation room staff know what to do if a major vascular injury happens. When confronted with this situation, immediately inform the anesthesiologist, the scrub nurse, and the remaining staff; inform the operating room coordinator; keep the operating room team updated; ask for help from another surgeon (vascular surgeon if available); inform the blood bank for crossmatching (at least 6 units); get fresh frozen plasma and platelets as required; get 0 Rh units; assure two large-bore cannulas for intravenous access; initiate antibiotic prophylaxis; keep the patient warm; prepare for open surgery (the scrub nurse is responsible for the vascular set) [5]. All these actions must be performed by nurses and runners, while both the surgeon and the anesthesiologist assess the vascular injury and the blood loss, apply pressure on the bleeding site while trying to control the hemorrhage, and decide what to do next. Victoria Asfour, from the Imperial College of London, recommends resorting to a major vascular injury protocol. This protocol summarizes the roles to be played by the runners, the nurses, the anesthesiologist, and the surgeon into three groups of actions [5]. During the entire repair process, it is mandatory to maintain coordination between the surgeon–anesthesiologist–nurse–blood department [9].

To anticipate this stressful situation, a preoperative briefing is paramount. Before beginning the operation, the entire team must know what is going to be done and why, the steps of the procedure, the main risks, and how to act in case of major complications. The surgeon must inform and anticipate any unusual findings or actions. Stress must be prevented, and a preoperative briefing is one way of doing it.

Knowing who to call for help, if necessary, is a question that must be addressed before the start of any surgery. The entire staff must know who the person is. If available, a vascular surgeon should be called, but a fellow general surgeon is also a very good alternative. The number of surgeons with a great deal of experience in managing major vascular injuries during minimally invasive procedures is scarce [5]. So, ideally within this setting, you should call someone who has experience in different procedures of general surgery and vascular surgery.

9.4 Vascular Injury Repair

From the very first stage of the procedure, both the surgeon and the assistant must remain calm. Two questions must be immediately addressed by the surgeon:

- Can I identify and control the bleeding site laparoscopically?
- Can I repair it myself or will I need help?

Although vascular repair can be performed laparoscopically, conversion to open surgery can be mandatory to assure fast and effective bleeding control and to promote appropriate and safe repair. Conversion to open surgery must not be viewed as a failure. Calling another surgeon or vascular surgeon for help is paramount. Even if the surgeon can repair the injury by himself, "a fresh mind" and "a new set of eyes" will help bring anxiety levels down. Do not ever be afraid or ashamed of calling for help. Sharing the decision process with another fellow is crucial for successfully treating a major complication.

Globally, there are three principals to perform a vascular repair:

- Proximal and distal vascular control (bleeding control).
- Exposure of the vessel and the injury (dissect the vessel if necessary).
- Repair with a non-absorbable suture.

It is very important to have good exposure before attempting to repair a vascular injury [5]. Placing a suture or a clamp with poor exposure can cause more damage or additional injuries to other structures. However, additional dissection of large vessels should be avoided if good injury exposure is already present [10].

9.4.1 How to Do It?

In the presence of a vascular injury during a PRA, there are a few procedures that must be followed to promote safe and efficient repair [1]. The steps outlined below overlap during the decision-making process.

1. The available working space is very limited and makes it difficult to perform a laparoscopic suture.

   This must be considered when deciding whether to convert or not to open surgery. Trocar positioning in a PRA is associated with limited freedom of the instruments and increases "sword fighting," making it difficult to perform a vascular suture [4].

2. Assess severity and nature of the injury.

   Although good injury exposure is mandatory, large vessel dissection should be avoided when not necessary [10]. It is very important to resist the temptation to blindly place clips or clamps. Doing this without good visualization of the injured vessel can result in more damage (vascular and collateral). Always take into account that a vein is harder to repair than an artery, and also that the "hemostatic suture" is not appropriate to repair a major vessel [5].

3. Can you repair it yourself?

   Even if you can repair it, asking for help is mandatory. If possible, call a vascular surgeon or ask for assistance from a fellow general surgeon [5].

4. Decide if immediate conversion is the best option for safe and efficient vascular repair.

   A surgeon's expertise and skills in laparoscopic suturing and vascular repair are crucial to decision-making. All surgeons must be able to perform a vascular repair during an inadvertent vascular accident.

5. Laparoscopically apply pressure with a gauze.

   Immediately place a gauze through the balloon trocar and apply pressure on the bleeding site. This is the fastest, simplest, and easiest way to control bleeding [5]. This action will give the surgical team and operating room staff time to think and prepare for repair.

6. Keep pneumoretroperitoneum pressure high.

   PRA allows for the use of high pressures of CO_2. This will help tamponade venous hemorrhage and give us a dry working space [1–3]. Retroperitoneoscopic adrenalectomy is performed with pressures up to 25 mmHg, which can help stop bleeding. Some authors recommend increasing the pressure up to 30 mmHg to obtain temporary hemostasis [4]. High pressure can cause gas embolism and cardiac instability. However, several studies have not reported a single case of pulmonary embolism or deep vein thrombosis (iliac or femoral) [3–11].

7. Place the patient in a Trendelenburg position.

   Some authors recommend the Trendelenburg as the preferred position in the presence of a major vascular injury. It decreases the venous pressure in the lower extremities and will keep brain cells irrigated in case of hypovolemia [5–12].

8. Use a fourth trocar.

   This extra port can be used for better tissue retraction and bleeding vessel exposure. It can also be used to place a laparoscopic vascular clamp if necessary [1].

9. Laparoscopic suture for vascular repair.

   Use a nonabsorbable polypropylene 000/0000 suture. Vessel stenosis must be avoided and therefore, separate stitches are to be preferred to continuous suture. Manipulate the vessel wall carefully. Smooth movements using a good needle holder are crucial for good repair. Pass the needle through the vessel wall and open the needle holder. Next, grab the needle tip and pull it carefully. This will help avoid vessel wall laceration.

10. Reduce pressure and inspect for hemostasis.

    High pneumoretroperitoneum pressure can give a false sense of security after a vascular repair. Bleeding recurrence can occur after deflation. Decrease pressure to 5 mmHg and inspect for hemostasis [2]. If there is no bleeding, the repair is finished.

11. Local hemostatic.

    Topical agents like fibrin, synthetic glues, and adhesives have proved their value as hemostatic and sealants [5]. Following a major vascular repair, these agents can be used to reinforce the repair [12].

12. Place a drain.

The retroperitoneal space is a virtual one, and tamponade will occur after deflation. Placing a drain will not avoid recurrence but will eventually help in its early diagnosis.

9.5 Vascular Injuries and Learning Curve

The learning curve is a key point of all surgical procedures. Knowing how many procedures surgeons should perform until they properly master it is a matter of constant debate. In our point of view, the learning curve is influenced by surgeons' experience in different procedures and the skills they have gained while performing different surgical techniques. The learning curve will be influenced by the surgeons themselves and similarly, they also represent a factor with an impact on the complication rate.

Rassweiller et al. demonstrate the importance of the learning curve. In the first 50 retroperitoneoscopic procedures (renal and adrenal), there was a 14% rate of complications, contrasting with a 2% complication rate in procedures 150-200. Additionally, conversion to open surgery decreased from 10% in the first 50 procedures to 4% in the procedures 150–200 [13]. Kumar et al. report a decrease in minor complications as more retroperitoneoscopic surgical procedures (renal and adrenal) are performed, although the number of major complications remains stable [2]. In the Meraney et al., analysis of 404 retroperitoneoscopic procedures (renal and adrenal) conversion to open surgery was not necessary for the last 200 procedures. This data reflects the impact of the learning curve [1]. In Essen, Alesina et al. report an operation time of 117 minutes during the learning phase for PRA. After performing 2310 PRA, they reduced operation time to 45 minutes and complication rate to less than 1% [4]. With increased experience, comes a decrease in the complication rate [2].

Gaining experience in the management of major vascular injuries during retroperitoneoscopic adrenalectomy is not easy because they are rare [2]. In 2006, Walz presented his results of 560 PRA performed on 520 patients. There was not a single case of major vascular injury. In fact, there were no cases of major bleeding in 11 conversions (2.0%). Walz only reports one case of reoperation due to bleeding from the gland remnant after partial adrenalectomy [3]. In 2019, Alesina reported no major vascular injuries after 2310 procedures [4]. In a case series analysis of the first 20 procedures performed by the author, one IVC injury was reported. Conversion to posterior open for a safe and effective vascular repair was necessary (see case report below) [14].

The rarity of major vascular injuries during PRA supports its safety. Moreover, there is no solid experience on how to manage these life-threatening complications. Injury to the IVC (including retro hepatic) is a possibility when dissecting the right gland and the right adrenal vein. An injury at this site is difficult to approach. Gaining experience in such a rare situation is not easy but performing other different surgical procedures can give you the skills you need. A surgeon should have experience in vascular surgery in order to know the principles of a vascular repair and be able to perform it. In a stressful situation like an IVC bleeding, a vascular surgeon may not be available. Additionally, many of them will also not have experience in managing a retro hepatic IVC injury. It is even more difficult to find someone with experience in laparoscopic vascular repair.

How can surgeons gain experience in the management of a retroperitoneal IVC injury? Trauma patients can be a learning site. However, retroperitoneal vascular injuries are rare. A Level 1 Trauma Center in the United States treated 65 IVC injuries and 39 abdominal aorta injuries due to blunt and penetrating trauma over a 10-year period [8]. Some of the patients had both aortic and IVC injuries. Suture was the most frequently used technique. Of course, all patients were treated by an open approach. In that analysis, the authors concluded that suprarenal located injury has a 15 times higher risk of mortality [8]. This is a common location of IVC injury during a PRA.

It is difficult for surgeons to learn how to deal with IVC injury just from severe trauma patients with a retroperitoneal vascular injury. Firstly, they are rare situations. Secondly, a surgeon must know what to do before facing a major vascular trauma in the emergency department. Active learning from books and videos can help doctors prepare for dealing with a major vascular injury. Periodic hands-on courses in animal models will also help surgeons to learn how to approach and repair these difficult located injuries [9]. Simulation and eventually digital/virtual constructed scenarios will be the future of a surgeon's learning process, like in airplane pilot training.

9.6   Case Report

In 2018, we had to treat a major vascular complication while performing a right PRA. It was an IVC injury. This report aims to share that experience and the difficulties a surgeon must deal with while managing a major vascular injury by posterior RA.

Firstly, stay calm. This is of paramount importance for a successful repair. Secondly, ask for immediate help from another surgeon. A "fresh mind" is crucial for a good repair. Thirdly, inform the anesthesiologist of what is happening and what you are about to do. Fourth, the scrub nurse and remaining operation room staff must immediately provide the required instruments to perform the repair. Fifth, do not hesitate to convert to open surgery if necessary. When the goal is fast bleeding control and vascular repair, conversion must not be seen as a failure but as a way to achieve that goal.

A male patient complaining of right lumbar pain was diagnosed with a giant (11 cm) nonfunctioning adrenal cyst. Abdominal Computed Tomography (CT) and Magnetic Resonance Imaging (MRI) were both performed to obtain detailed anatomical information (Figs. 9.1 and 9.2). He had no comorbidities. Despite the large size of the lesion, the surgical team decided to use the posterior RA. The plan was to dissect the cyst as much as possible without rupture, aspirate its liquid content, ligate the adrenal vein, and retrieve it in a bag. This was not the first time this approach was performed on a lesion this size.

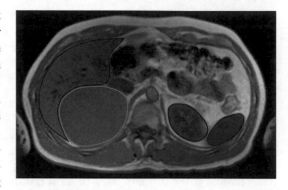

Fig. 9.1 MRI—axial plane. An 11-cm giant cyst of the right adrenal gland (*yellow*) is pushing the right lobe of the liver (*light brown*). The cyst pushes and flattens the IVC (*blue*). Aorta (*red*). Left kidney (*dark brown*). Spleen (*purple*)

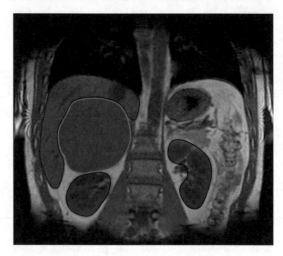

Fig. 9.2 MRI—coronal plane. The giant cyst of the right adrenal (*yellow*) is pushing the right kidney (*dark brown*) down. The liver (*light brown*) is also pushed and compressed by the huge lesion

Although minimally invasive surgery has several advantages over open surgery, it has a possible negative impact on R0 resection and a higher risk of cystic rupture. This is the rationality for advising open surgery for lesions larger than 6 cm or suspected of harboring cancer (see Chap. 5) [14, 15]. However, minimally invasive surgery has been used for large lesions. In 2016, we successfully resected a 14-cm cystic pheochromocytoma by posterior RA [15].

After placing the trocars as usual (see Chap. 7) and setting the pneumoretroperitoneum to 25 mmHg, the cystic lesion was immediately

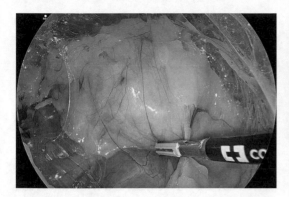

Fig. 9.3 Cyst with 11 cm over the upper pole of the right kidney. It occupies the entire operation field and pushes the kidney down

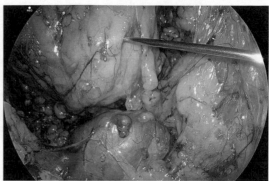

Fig. 9.4 Aspiration of the cystic content with a Veress needle. This was crucial to give the surgeon working space to go on with dissection

identified due to its large size (Fig. 9.3). Dissection started with LigaSure® from lateral to medial, separating the cyst from the upper pole of the kidney. Identification of the IVC was the next step and it was done uneventfully. At this time, dissection could not go further due to the large size of the cyst. Aspiration of its liquid content was performed using a Veress needle and a laparoscopic aspirator (Fig. 9.4). Clear serous fluid was aspirated. Dissection resumed even though the cyst was not fully empty. The cystic lesion was separated from the IVC with blunt dissection, but the adrenal vein was not immediately found. The surgical team decided to proceed with dissection all around the lesion, freeing the cyst as much as possible from the surrounding structures. An accidental opening of the cyst occurred, which completely emptied the lesion but also facilitated the procedure. A short adrenal vein was finally found and ligated with the LigaSure®. At this point, the cyst was only fixed to the IVC by a dense adhesion.

During the final dissection, a small injury to the IVC occurred when using the LigaSure®. It was a small hole with a size of approximately 2 mm (Fig. 9.5). No significant bleeding occurred due to the high pressure of the pneumoretroperitoneum (25 mmHg). A gauze was immediately introduced through the balloon trocar and pressure was applied on the injury site for fast bleeding control (Fig. 9.6). This gave the entire team time to prepare for vascular repair, as well as time for another surgeon to arrive.

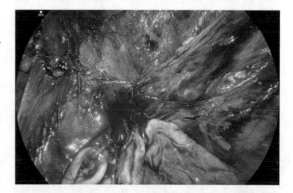

Fig. 9.5 A small IVC injury. No significant bleeding due to the 25-mmHg pneumoretroperitoneum

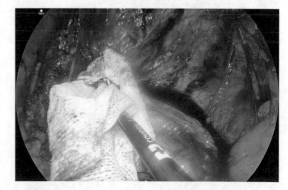

Fig. 9.6 Applying pressure with a gauze on the injury site is the fastest and easiest way to achieve temporary bleeding control. It gives the surgical team time to prepare for definitive repair

Since the IVC injury was easily identified and visualization was good, we decided to perform a laparoscopic vascular repair with a Prolene®

0000 (Fig. 9.7). No fourth trocar was placed. However, due to the positioning of the trocars, we struggled with "sword fighting." After several attempts, no-stitch was performed. The camera was changed to the balloon trocar and the medial trocar was used as a working port to try to increase the angle of the instruments and overtake the "sword fighting." We managed to get the first stitch, but when an attempt was made on the second knot, the vein tore even more (Fig. 9.8). At this point, the surgical team decided to convert to open posterior surgery.

While keeping the patient in the same position, a lumbar incision below the 12th rib was made. After entering the retroperitoneum, the assistant had to strongly pull the patient's ribs with a retractor to give the surgeon enough working space. Blood was now covering the entire operation field. Pressure on the bleeding site was applied with gauze, and the blood was then aspirated to give the surgeon a dry operation field. By gently retrieving the gauze, the IVC injury was identified. It was not in an easy-to-access position. The surgeon managed to repair the injury with a noncontinuous suture of Prolene 0000 (two stitches). No vascular clamp was used, nor was additional IVC dissection necessary since injury boundaries were readily visible. A hemostatic sponge (TachoSil®) was placed covering the suture and a drain was left in the retroperitoneum. The incision was sutured.

The patient spent 1 day in the Intensive Care Unit (ICU) and was then transferred to the surgery ward. The first oral intake was on postoperative day two. The drain was removed on day three (<50 ml). The patient was discharged home on the fifth postoperative day. Three months after surgery, the patient was recovering successfully, without pain and only complained of mild hypoesthesia on the lateral abdominal wall. He returned to his normal activity without impairments.

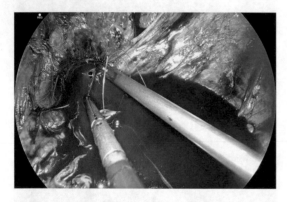

Fig. 9.7 Suturing the IVC injury by posterior RA

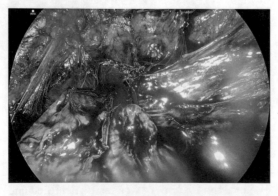

Fig. 9.8 IVC tore even more while performing retroperitoneoscopic vascular repair. The vein wall is fragile, and "sword fighting" makes it very difficult to suture

References

1. Meraney AM, Samee AA-E, Gill IS. Vascular and bowel complications during retroperitoneal laparoscopic surgery. J Urol. 2002;168(5):1941–4.
2. Kumar M, Kumar R, Hemal AK, Gupta NP. Complications of retroperitoneoscopic surgery at one centre. BJU Int. 2001;87(7):607–12.
3. Walz MK, Alesina PF, Wenger FA, Deligiannis A, Szuczik E, Petersenn S, et al. Posterior retroperitoneoscopic adrenalectomy-results of 560 procedures in 520 patients. Surgery. 2006;140(6):943–8.
4. Alesina PF. Retroperitoneal adrenalectomy-learning curve, practical tips and tricks, what limits its wider uptake. Gland Surg. 2019;8(Suppl 1):S36–40.
5. Asfour V, Smythe E, Attia R. Vascular injury at laparoscopy: a guide to management. J Obstet Gynaecol. 2018;38(5):598–606.
6. Baggish MS. Analysis of 31 cases of major-vessel injury associated with gynecologic laparoscopy operations. J Gynecol Surg. 2003;19(2):63–73.
7. Burkitt HG, Young B, Heath JW. Sistema Circulatório. In: Wheater's functional histology: a text and colour atlas. Third Edition. 1994. p. 140–52.
8. Coimbra R, Hoyt DB, Winchell R, Simons R, Fortlage D, Garcia J. The ongoing challenge of retroperitoneal vascular injuries. Am J Surg. 1996;172(5):541–4.

9. Costa Almeida CE. Retroperitoneal vascular injuries. Did something change? [Internet]. Surgical Thoughts: A blog about surgery. 2020 [cited 2022 Jan 5]. https://carloscostaalmeida.wixsite.com/surgicalthoughts/

10. Pereira BMT, Chiara O, Ramponi F, Weber DG, Cimbanassi S, de Simone B, et al. WSES position paper on vascular emergency surgery. World J Emerg Surg. 2015;10:49.

11. Cabalag MS, Mann GB, Gorelik A, Miller JA. Posterior retroperitoneoscopic adrenalectomy: outcomes and lessons learned from initial 50 cases. ANZ J Surg. 2015;85(6):478–82.

12. Pappa E, Evangelopoulos DS, Benetos IS, Pnevmaticos S. Vascular injury in elective ante-rior surgery of the lumbar spine: a narrative review. Cureus. 2021;13(12):e20267.

13. Rassweiler JJ, Seemann O, Frede T, Henkel TO, Alken P. Retroperitoneoscopy: experience with 200 cases. J Urol. 1998;160(4):1265–9.

14. Costa Almeida CE, Caroço T, Silva MA, Baião JM, Costa A, Albano MN, et al. An update of posterior retroperitoneoscopic adrenalectomy—case series. Int J Surg Case Rep. 2020;71:120–5.

15. Costa Almeida CE, Silva M, Carvalho L, Costa Almeida CM. Adrenal giant cystic pheochromocy-toma treated by posterior retroperitoneoscopic adre-nalectomy. Int J Surg Case Rep. 2017;30:201–4.

Converting to Open Surgery

10

Oscar Vidal, Martí Manyalich Blasi,
and David Saavedra-Perez

10.1 Introduction

Adrenal masses are one of the most prevalent human tumors. Its incidence is approximately 3% in middle age and increases to 10% in the elderly [1]. In this sense, laparoscopic adrenalectomy (LAdr) has become the gold standard for the treatment of adrenal diseases in recent decades [2]. Two alternative surgical methodologies are currently promoted: the transperitoneal laparoscopic approach (TLA) and the posterior retroperitoneoscopic adrenalectomy (PRA) [3]. Interestingly, most adrenalectomy procedures during the early and mid-1990s were performed using an open approach. According to the study by Murphy et al., from 1998 to 2006, the number of adrenal resections in the United States increased significantly from 3241 to 5019 cases, and the majority (83%) of adrenalectomies were performed using an open approach. Currently, the surgeon's increased experience, advanced laparoscopic techniques, improved technology, and better short-term patient outcomes have led to laparoscopy displacing open surgery, making LAdr the procedure of choice in most cases [4].

However, LAdr shows some complications, with a reported overall complication rate of approximately 10% (range 2.9–20), with bleeding being the most prevalent complication. Organ injury, including damage to the liver, spleen, pancreas, kidney, large bowel, and diaphragm, has also been observed [5, 6]. Nevertheless, several studies have reported that LAdr has greater benefits in terms of patient outcomes, decreasing postoperative pain and disability, length of hospital stay, complication rate, and blood loss compared to open surgery. In addition, LAdr allows patients to return to normal activity faster [5, 7].

Despite the advantages of laparoscopic approach (LA) and the fact that there are no contraindications to LAdr, the review study by Assalia and Gagner indicates that the mean conversion rate is 3.6% (range 0–12) [6]. Several factors may increase the risk of open conversion, giving a less encouraging scenario. Identification of these risk factors would improve preoperative stratification, patient safety, and postoperative expectations, enhancing the cost-benefit balance and giving a better perspective to the medical team.

O. Vidal · M. Manyalich Blasi (✉)
D. Saavedra-Perez
General & Digestive Surgery Department, ICMDIM,
Hospital Clinic Barcelona, IDIBAPS, University of
Barcelona, Barcelona, Spain
e-mail: ovidal@clinic.cat;
manyalich@clinic.cat; dsaavedr@clinic.cat

© The Author(s), under exclusive license to Springer Nature Switzerland AG 2023
C. E. Costa Almeida (ed.), *Posterior Retroperitoneoscopic Adrenalectomy*,
https://doi.org/10.1007/978-3-031-19995-0_10

The aim of this chapter is to discuss the risk factors that determine when and how to convert LA to open surgery.

10.2 Definition of Conversion to Open Surgery

Conversion to open surgery has been defined as an abdominal wall incision larger than 5 cm performed to make other manipulations different from specimen retrieval. In general, the conversion rate is expected to decrease as the laparoscopist experience level increases. However, some causes for conversion to open surgery even when there is sufficient experience include difficult dissection, severe bleeding, injuries to adjacent organs or tissues, risk for tumor rupture, inadequate intraperitoneal insufflations, and inability to identify the target lesion [8].

10.3 Risk Factors Associated with Conversion to Open Surgery during Transperitoneal Laparoscopic Adrenalectomy

Variables such as age, American Society of Anesthesiologists (ASA) physical status classification, sex, previous abdominal surgery, and laterality have not been related to the necessity for conversion from laparoscopic to open adrenalectomy. In addition, although right-sided tumors have been reported to be more predisposed to bleeding because of the short adrenal vein draining immediately to the inferior vena cava (IVC), in some studies, it has not been associated with the conversion to open surgery [8, 9].

On the other hand, several studies have associated risk factors such as obesity (body mass index (BMI) ≥ 30 kg/m^2), large adrenal masses (tumors >5 cm in diameter), and pheochromocytoma, with conversion to open surgery [8, 9]. Therefore, the proper selection of patients and identification of their associated risk factors are crucial.

10.3.1 Obesity

The association between obesity and conversion to open adrenalectomy is based on the difficulty of dissection, difficult cannula placement, difficult anatomical visualization due to excessive intraperitoneal fat, difficult instrument manipulation through an excessively thick abdominal wall, and longer operating time, which may result in an increased risk of major bleeding and other complications. In addition, morbid obesity may require high intra-abdominal insufflation pressure to establish an adequate working space, and high-pressure pneumoperitoneum may impede venous return [9].

Therefore, transperitoneal approaches (anterior and lateral) or the use of longer instruments are better choices than retroperitoneal approaches when there are large adrenal masses. However, the retroperitoneal approach seems to be better in small adrenal masses in obese patients [9, 10]. In addition, laparoscopic ultrasound can be helpful for locating the left adrenal vein, especially when it is obscured by a large amount of retroperitoneal fat, helping some obese patients to be candidates for LAdr (TLA or PRA) [11].

10.3.2 Size of the Tumor

The size of the tumor has been found to be the most important predictor of conversion. A large tumor will have a distended retroperitoneal vasculature due to compression, thus increasing the risk of bleeding. The growth of the adrenal tumor also causes reorganization of the surrounding tissues, making the tumor more difficult to excise, which leads to prolonging the time required for the surgical procedure [8, 9]. Although tumors larger than 5 cm are a risk factor for conversion, there is no consensus about which size of adrenal tumor is appropriate for an open or a LA. It has been reported that some surgeons laparoscopically resect adrenal tumors up to 15 cm in size [12]. In those cases, the use of laparoscopic ultrasound imaging may have been helpful and may have reduced conversions. Ultrasound helps to define the relationship of tumors to adjacent structures, identifying the adrenal vein for direct dissection (especially for left-sided lesions), confirming the presence of pathology, and the resectability of large masses [11, 13].

Furthermore, some researchers have used the size of the adrenal tumor to predict the risk of malignancy. Adrenal tumors >5–6 cm in size have been found to have a high risk of malignancy (between 35% and 98%) [12].

10.3.3 Pheochromocytoma

Pheochromocytomas are catecholamine-producing tumors derived from chromaffin cells of the adrenal medulla [14]. The feasibility and efficacy of LAdr in cases of pheochromocytoma have been extensively confirmed, but patients with pheochromocytoma had significantly higher perioperative complication rates than those with benign, non-pheochromocytoma tumors [15].

There are several concerns about the LAdr to treat pheochromocytoma due to the potential hemodynamic effects of catecholamine secretion, which can induce malignant hypertension in the initial pneumoperitoneum or during minimal traction on surrounding tissues [16]. Likewise, the occurrence of both hypertensive and hypotensive intraoperative episodes during the same procedure has been reported [14].

LAdr (TLA and PRA) in patients with pheochromocytoma has been associated with a higher incidence of conversion to an open procedure [8]. Therefore, it has been suggested that in cases where a large pheochromocytoma (>5–7 cm) is observed, as well as in cases of difficult dissection, invasion, adhesions, and the need for preoperative hospitalization, patients may be more likely to require open adrenalectomy or a conversion to an open approach [14, 17, 18]. Understandably, the need for conversion was associated with increased intraoperative hypertensive episodes, increased mean operative time, mean anesthesia duration, postoperative complications, and length of stay [14].

However, enhanced anesthetic and laparoscopic techniques, as well as perioperative patient optimization, have significantly improved perioperative outcomes, with low conversion (<10%) and morbidity rates (<20%) [14].

10.4 How to Convert?

There are different incision options for open adrenalectomy approach when converting is required: median supraumbilical laparotomy, subcostal laparotomy, modified Makuuchi incision ("J"), and thoracoabdominal incision (also see Chap. 3).

A posterior approach can also be performed with the patient in a prone position through a curvilinear incision that runs from the ipsilateral paramedian line and extending laterally. This approach requires removal of rib 12 to extensively expose the retroperitoneal space. The remainder of the operation proceeds similarly to an endoscopic retroperitoneal adrenalectomy.

10.4.1 Choice of Incision

Several factors must be considered when deciding on the type of incision:

1. Size of the tumor and need for concomitant resection (e.g., nephrectomy or hepatectomy, anatomical or not), or vascular reconstruction.
2. Tumor location and direction of invasion.
3. Existing patient position during conversion of a minimally invasive procedure.

10.4.2 Open Right Adrenalectomy

The modified right Makuuchi or modified subcostal incision is the preferred incision because they provide adequate exposure for safe dissection. The right lobe of the liver needs to be fully mobilized by dividing the triangular ligament, while moving the liver superomedially to expose the infrahepatic and retrohepatic IVC, as well as the retrocaval collateral vessels.

10.4.3 Open Left Adrenalectomy

Typically, this operation is performed through a left subcostal or "J" incision on the left side. A midline supraumbilical laparotomy can be performed, but this incision may be insufficient for proper exposure.

10.5 Concluding Remarks

LAdr is a safe and effective procedure with significant advantages over the open procedure. Careful selection of surgical candidates should be based on both patient and tumor factors, given that patients with more comorbidities, obesity, large tumor sizes, and pheochromocytoma are at risk for conversion to open adrenalectomy and increased perioperative complications [15]. However, conversion to open surgery as well as the open approach should not be considered a failure. The surgeon should not hesitate to convert to an open procedure or indicate that the best procedure is an open approach, considering that open adrenalectomy is a perfect solution in cases of adrenalectomies with different associated risk factors. In addition, the preoperative analysis can assess the risk of conversion, which will lead to better planning of laparoscopic surgery. Thus, with the help of an accurate prediction, patients can also be fully informed to take the measures they deem appropriate [8, 9].

References

1. Mansmann G, Lau J, Balk E, Rothberg M, Miyachi Y, Bornstein SR. The clinically inapparent adrenal mass: update in diagnosis and management. Endocr Rev. 2004;25(2):309–40.
2. Carr AA, Wang TS. Minimally invasive adrenalectomy. Surg Oncol Clin N Am. 2016;25(1):139–52.
3. Kozłowski T, Choromanska B, Wojskowicz P, Astapczyk K, Łukaszewicz J, Rutkowski D, et al. Laparoscopic adrenalectomy: lateral transperitoneal versus posterior retroperitoneal approach – prospective randomized trial. Wideochirurgia I Inne Tech Maloinwazyjne. 2019;14(2):160–9.
4. Murphy MM, Witkowski ER, Ng SC, McDade TP, Hill JS, Larkin AC, et al. Trends in adrenalectomy: a recent national review. Surg Endosc. 2010;24(10):2518–26.
5. Gaujoux S, Bonnet S, Leconte M, Zohar S, Bertherat J, Bertagna X, et al. Risk factors for conversion and complications after unilateral laparoscopic adrenalectomy. Br J Surg. 2011;98(10):1392–9.
6. Assalia A, Gagner M. Laparoscopic adrenalectomy. Br J Surg. 2004;91(10):1259–74.
7. Hazzan D, Shiloni E, Golijanin D, Jurim O, Gross D, Reissman P. Laparoscopic vs open adrenalectomy for benign adrenal neoplasm: a comparative study. Surg Endosc. 2001;15(11):1356–8.
8. Vidal O, Saavedra-Perez D, Martos JM, de la Quintana A, Rodriguez JI, Villar J, et al. Risk factors for open conversion of lateral transperitoneal laparoscopic adrenalectomy: retrospective cohort study of the Spanish Adrenal Surgery Group (SASG). Surg Endosc. 2020;34(8):3690–5.
9. Shen ZJ, Chen SW, Wang S, Jin XD, Chen J, Zhu Y, et al. Predictive factors for open conversion of laparoscopic adrenalectomy: a 13-year review of 456 cases. J Endourol. 2007;21(11):1333–7.
10. Lezoche E, Guerrieri M, Feliciotti F, Paganini AM, Perretta S, Baldarelli M, et al. Anterior, lateral, and posterior retroperitoneal approaches in endoscopic adrenalectomy. Surg Endosc Other Interv Tech. 2002;16(1):96–9.
11. Lucas SW, Spitz JD, Arregui ME. The use of intraoperative ultrasound in laparoscopic adrenal surgery: the Saint Vincent experience. Surg Endosc. 1999;13(11):1093–8.
12. Kebebew E, Siperstein AE, Clark OH, Duh QY. Results of laparoscopic adrenalectomy for suspected and unsuspected malignant adrenal neoplasms. Arch Surg. 2002;137(8):948–53.
13. Pautler SE, Choyke PL, Pavlovich CP, Daryanani K, Walther MM. Intraoperative ultrasound aids in dissection during laparoscopic partial adrenalectomy. J Urol. 2002;168(4 Pt 1):1352–5.
14. Schweitzer ML, Nguyen-Thi PL, Mirallie E, Vriens M, Raffaelli M, Klein M, et al. Conversion during laparoscopic adrenalectomy for pheochromocytoma: a cohort study in 244 patients. J Surg Res. 2019;243:309–15.
15. Chen Y, Scholten A, Chomsky-Higgins K, Nwaogu I, Gosnell JE, Seib C, et al. Risk factors associated with perioperative complications and prolonged length of stay after laparoscopic adrenalectomy. JAMA Surg. 2018;153(11):1036–41.
16. Kalady MF, McKinlay R, Olson JA, Pinheiro J, Lagoo S, Park A, et al. Laparoscopic adrenalectomy for pheochromocytoma: a comparison to aldosteronoma and incidentaloma. Surg Endosc Other Interv Tech. 2004;18(4):621–5.
17. Shen WT, Sturgeon C, Clark OH, Duh QY, Kebebew E. Should pheochromocytoma size influence surgical approach? A comparison of 90 malignant and 60 benign pheochromocytomas. Surgery. 2004;136(6):1129–37.
18. Inabnet WB, Pitre J, Bernard D, Chapuis Y. Comparison of the hemodynamic parameters of open and laparoscopic adrenalectomy for pheochromocytoma. World J Surg. 2000;24(5):574–8.

Final Outcomes

11

Carlos Eduardo Costa Almeida and Teresa Vieira Caroço

11.1 Introduction

The first laparoscopic adrenalectomy was described in 1992 by Higashihara [1], from Japan, and Gagner [2], from Canada. This description followed the emerging use of minimally invasive surgery since the early 1980s [3]. After 1992, endoscopic surgery became the gold standard for benign adrenal lesions [4–6]. The reduced aggressiveness of laparoscopic surgery, with less postoperative pain and faster recovery, combined with the augmented reality image that improved the visualization of anatomical structures, promoted the dissemination of minimally invasive approaches. New approaches emerged with the minimally invasive surgery revolution. In 1994, the retroperitoneal adrenalectomy was described in Japan by Uchida [7], in Sweden by Johansson [8], and in New Zeeland by Whittle [9].

Posterior retroperitoneoscopic adrenalectomy (PRA) was developed and extensively studied by Martin Walz from Essen. In 2001, Martin Walz standardized the technique after a five-year experience and 143 procedures [10]. Since then, PRA

has gained worldwide acceptance [3] because it is a safe and feasible technique [3, 4, 5, 10, 11].

Final outcomes are crucial to evaluate the success of a technique. Operative time, complication rate, blood loss, conversion rate, postoperative pain, in-hospital days, return to normal activity, mortality rate, and learning curve are all factors with impact on the referral and acceptance of a surgical technique.

PRA soon demonstrated its several advantages over anterior and lateral transperitoneal laparoscopic adrenalectomy (TLAdr). Due to its direct access to the gland without incursion into the peritoneal cavity, PRA is not only fast and easy to perform but also eliminates the risk of incidental injury to abdominal viscera [4, 5, 12]. It has lower operative time, less postoperative pain, less blood loss, lower morbidity, shorter in-hospital length of stay, and a faster return to normal activity [3, 4, 5, 12, 13]. Additionally, PRA promotes a faster return of bowel movements and has a better cosmetic result [5, 11].

Despite PRA advantages, TLAdr is mostly used because it is safe, has a short learning curve, and is a standardized procedure. In the transperitoneal approach, the surgeon works in the peritoneal cavity, with which all surgeons are familiarized. This is one of the main reasons why many surgeons keep using the anterior transperitoneal approach. Another reason is the lack of anatomical landmarks at the beginning of the procedure, which gives the PRA-initiating sur-

C. E. Costa Almeida (✉)
General Surgery, Portuguese Oncology Institute of Coimbra, Hospital CUF Coimbra, Coimbra, Portugal
e-mail: carloscostaalmeida@yahoo.com

T. V. Caroço
General Surgery Department, Portuguese Oncology Institute of Coimbra, Coimbra, Portugal

© The Author(s), under exclusive license to Springer Nature Switzerland AG 2023
C. E. Costa Almeida (ed.), *Posterior Retroperitoneoscopic Adrenalectomy*,
https://doi.org/10.1007/978-3-031-19995-0_11

geon the false idea of extreme difficulty [5, 14]. However, nowadays, PRA is a safe, feasible, and standardized approach. That is why some surgeons have already changed from TLAdr to PRA [12]. Another advantage of the retroperitoneoscopic approach (RA) when compared to the laparoscopic one is the lower effect insufflating the retroperitoneum has on the patients' hemodynamic and respiratory parameters [12]. However, surgeons must not insufflate the retroperitoneum too fast. Insufflation must be gentle. One of our patients had sudden asystole when the retroperitoneum was insufflated to 25 mmHg. In such cases, immediate chaos can arise because the patient is prone position, precluding efficient resuscitation maneuvers. Deinsufflation immediately reverted the asystole. Following a slow insufflation up to 25 mmHg, the surgery went uneventfully [5, 12, 15].

Learning the technique with an experienced surgeon is paramount. There are tips and tricks that will help surgeons easily perform PRA (see Chap. 7). Surgeons must change from the anterior anatomical to the posterior perspective. Changing their mindset is crucial to understand the anatomy from this "back door" approach [16]. Identifying the upper pole of the kidney within the perirenal fat is technically challenging. However, it is key to the learning curve [12, 15]. Having experience in other fields of laparoscopic surgery is another factor with a positive impact on surgeons' performance when starting PRA [5].

11.2　Operative Time

Operative time is not the most important outcome. One surgical procedure is not better than another just because it is faster. However, if a surgical technique can treat the same disease with the same results in a safe, faster, and feasible way, that technique should become the gold standard.

In 2001, Martin Walz (Essen, Germany) reported an operative time of 101 ± 39 min after the first 143 procedures. From these, 23 PRA (17%) were performed in less than 1 h [10]. The

same group from Essen was able to decrease the mean operative time to 45 min after 2310 procedures performed between 1994 and 2018 [3]. In a retrospective analysis of 560 PRA, Walz et al. reported a median operative time of 55 min and a mean operative time of 67 ± 40 min. However, if those 560 procedures are divided into five progressive groups of 112, a gradual reduction in operative time is made evident. The first 112 procedures had a mean operative time of 106 min, while the last 112 had a mean operative time of 40 min ($p < 0,001$). There was no difference in tumor size among the groups [4]. Operative time decreased as surgeons' experience increased.

Other authors reported different operative times. Kiriakopoulos had a mean operative time of 105.6 min for PRA, which was lower than for TLAdr [17]. In 2015, Porpiglia, from Italy, reported a mean operative time of 90 min [18]. Also in 2015, Cabalag presented a mean operative time of 70.5 min after 50 PRA. In this analysis, there was a statistically significant reduction in operative time in the first 15 procedures [12]. Barczynski, from Poland, reported a mean operative time of 50.8 min after 33 PRA [19]. A 2011 publication from the United States reported a mean operative time of 114 min, after successfully performing PRA in 118 cases of 125 scheduled [20]. Also from the USA, Nancy Perrier took a mean of 121 min to perform PRA in 62 patients [16] (Table 11.1).

In 2018, CE Costa Almeida analyzed his first 10 cases [5]. Mean operative time was 46.7 min (30–70 min) for lesions with a mean size of 4.1 cm, including one 14-cm cystic pheochromocytoma. Preoperative diagnoses were three pheochromocytomas, four Conns, two Cushings, and one nonfunctioning tumor. Two years later (2020), CE Costa Almeida published a comparative analysis between the first group and the second group of ten cases [15]. Mean operative time in the second group was 31.1 min, contrasting with the 46.7 min in the first group. This represented a significant reduction in operative time ($p = 0.036$). Both groups were equal in tumor size (a mean of 3.5 cm). Analyzing all patients, the mean operative time was 38.9 min, and a decrease in operative time was noted as more patients were

Table 11.1 Data from different case series of PRA published in worldwide literature. Mean tumor size was identical in all studies. Mean operative time was 38.9 min to 121 min. The largest case series presented a mean operative time of 45 min and morbidity <1%. Complications (0–16%) were mostly minor. After 20 PRA, CE Costa Almeida was able to reach a mean operative time of 38.9 min with 0% of postoperative complications. Blood loss was minimal in all studies. Mortality was 0% in all case series

	Walz 2006 [4]	Perrier 2008 [16]	Dickson 2011 [20]	Porpiglia 2014 [18]	Barczynski 2014 [19]	Kiriakopoulos 2015 [17]	Cabalag 2015 [12]	Bakkar 2017 [23]	Alesina 2018 [3]	CE Costa Almeida 2020 [15]
N	560	68	125	50	33	19	50	14	2310	20
Tumor size (cm)	2.9	3.4	2.7	N/A	3.9	3.7	N/A	3.3	N/A	3.5
Operative time (min)	67	121	114	90	50.8	105.6	70.5	87.5	45	38.9
Blood loss (ml)	10	N/A	14–18	50	52.7	N/A	N/A	N/A	N/A	20
Morbidity (%)	15.7	16	11.2	14	12.1[a]	N/A	8	0	<1	5
Minor (%)	14.4	–	–	–	12.1	–	–	–	–	0
Major (%)	1.3	–	–	–	–	–	–	–	–	5
Intraoperative (%)	–	–	2.4	2	–	–	0	–	–	5
Postoperative (%)	–	–	8.8	12	12.1	–	8	–	–	0
Conversion (%)	2	8.8	5.6	8	0	0	0	0	N/A	10
Posterior open (n)	7	–	–	0	–	–	–	–	–	1
Anterior open (n)	2	–	–	0	–	–	–	–	–	1
Lateral laparosc. (n)	2	–	–	0	–	–	–	–	–	0
Anterior laparosc. (n)	0	–	–	4	–	–	–	–	–	0
In-hospital days	N/A	3	N/A	N/A	2.9	2.1	1	3	N/A	1.7
Mortality (%)	0	0	0	0	0	0	0	0	0	0

N/A not available

[a]Considering as complications one pneumonia, one tachyarrhythmia, and two transient hypoesthesia of the abdominal wall. Excluded as complications two cases of subcutaneous emphysema

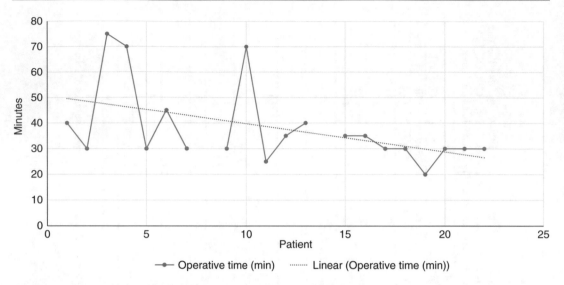

Fig. 11.1 Operative time evolution during 22 consecutive PRA performed by the first author. Operative time decreases with experience. Stabilization is noted after the first procedures

being operated on [15]. Figure 11.1 shows the evolution of the operative time during that period, evidencing a continuous decrease in operative time. After the first patients, operative time stabilized around 30 minutes, and with increasing experience, operative time decreased. With these results, PRA matched the operative times of laparoscopic cholecystectomy and endoscopic hernia repair [4].

Tumor type (pheochromocytoma, $p < 0,001$), tumor size >3 cm ($p < 0.05$), male ($p < 0,001$–0.05), complete versus partial resection ($p < 0.05$), and Body Mass Index (BMI) > 35, are factors that influence operative time [3, 7, 8, 20, 21]. According to the authors, operative time is also influenced by the surgeon's experience [15]. In 2006, Walz et al. found that operating the right-hand side implied longer operative time ($p < 0.05$) at the beginning of the learning curve. This was not evident in the last 200/560 procedures [4]. The reason for the increased operative time if operating on the right side might be the dissection near the inferior vena cava (IVC), and the need to dissect a small adrenal vein [20]. With experience, this dissection is carried out faster and more smoothly. The pronounced muscles in the male's flank can make it harder and require a longer time to perform the technique. To overcome this anatomical draw-back, accurate trocar placement is crucial. Obesity precludes the creation of good working space and increases operative time. Increasing the pneumoretroperitoneum up to 30 mmHg if BMI ≥35 can help to create a working space to successfully perform PRA [20]. Although not prohibitive, obesity makes the procedure extremely challenging due to the inability to appropriately expand the retroperitoneum, along with the difficult dissection created by the great amount of fat [16, 20]. Patients with a BMI >45 are not good candidates for PRA [4].

11.3 Complication Rate and Mortality

Complications in PRA are uncommon and mostly minor [22]. Possible complications are pleural tear, pneumothorax, surgical site infection, pneumonia, bleeding, relaxation, and/or hypoesthesia of abdominal wall (see Chap. 8). According to several studies, increasing experience results in a decrease in complication rate. Alesina reports a decrease in complication rate to less than 1% after 2310 procedures performed in Essen in a 24-year period [3]. Additionally, a 50% decrease in complication rate is possible as experience is gained [20].

In 2001, Martin Walz presented an intraoperative complication rate of 5%, and a postoperative complication rate of 13% after 143 procedures. All complications were minor [10]. In 2006, Walz reported a global complication rate of 15.7% (88/560 procedures). Major complications and minor complications after 560 PRA were 1.3% and 14.4%, respectively [4]. After performing 50 PRA, a group from Turin reported 2% and 12% of intraoperative and postoperative complications, respectively. Globally they had a total of seven (14%) complications [18]. Cabalag reported four postoperative complications (8%) following 50 PRA, including one temporary T12 neuropraxia [12]. From the USA, Dickson [20] reported an 11.2% and Perrier a 16% [16] complication rate. Following the first 10 cases, CE Costa Almeida reported a postoperative complication rate of 0% [5], and after performing 20 procedures, only one (5%) intraoperative complication (inferior vena cava injury), and no (0%) postoperative complication [15] (Table 11.1).

It is easy to understand that PRA has a low complication rate and that most complications are minor and temporary. Although decreasing with experience, the complication rate is typically low since the beginning of the learning curve. The mortality rate has been consistently reported as 0% [4, 5, 10, 12, 15, 17].

11.4 Conversion Rate and Blood Loss

Conversion must not be seen as a complication or a failure. The patient always comes first, and the surgeon must be comfortable with the need to change to another approach. Conversion rate varies in the literature. No conversion (0%) was reported by Kiriakopoulos [17] and Cabalag [12] after 19 and 50 procedures, respectively. Barczynski, from Poland, also reported 0% of conversions after 33 procedures [19]. On the other hand, Propiglia [18] reported a conversion to anterior laparoscopic approach in four cases (8%), and Dickson [20] converted 6.6% of his patients. A higher rate of conversion was reported in 2008 by Nancy Perrier, 8.8% [16].

In 2001, Martin Walz reported a conversion rate of 5% affecting 7 procedures out of 143, and a median blood loss of 54 ± 72 ml [10]. Five years later, in a total of 560 PRA for primary neoplasms, metastases (bronchial cancer, renal cancer, non-Hodgkin lymphoma), and ACTH-depending bilateral hyperplasia, Walz reported the need to convert to posterior open, anterior open, or lateral laparoscopic in only 11 procedures (2.0%)—four in left-sided and seven in right-sided disease. Conversion to posterior open occurred because of cardiac instability, failure to progress in Cushing syndromes, and technical difficulty. Anterior open was necessary because of dense adhesions in metastatic adrenals. Conversion to lateral laparoscopic was the option in severe obesity (BMI > 45) [4].

A conversion rate of 10% has been reported by the first author. Comparing the first group of 10 cases with the second group of 10 cases, conversion rate was the same, representing one patient in each group [13]. One patient was converted to anterior open because of extensive retroperitoneal fibrosis resulting from severe lumbar trauma some years before [5]. The other patient was converted to posterior open because of an inferior vena cava (IVC) injury. "Sword fighting" because of the acute angle the instruments are placed in, turned the vascular suture hard to perform, and conversion was the solution to control the bleeding.

Mean blood loss reported by Martin Walz after 549 non-converted PRA was 10 ml. Only one patient had to be transfused due to postoperative bleeding from the adrenal remnant after a partial adrenalectomy [4]. On the contrary, greater blood loss was reported by both Porpiglia [18] and Barczynski [19] in 2014, with a mean of 50 ml (20–210 ml) and 52.7 ml (34.4–71 ml), respectively. In 2018, CE Costa Almeida reported neglectable blood loss after the first 10 PRA performed for six left-sided tumors and four right-sided lesions [5]. In 2020, blood loss was around 20 ml following 20 PRA [15]. In conclusion, in most of the cases blood loss was neglectable (Table 11.1).´

11.5 Postoperative Pain

Postoperative pain evaluation is very subjective, and patients themselves are a bias. The need for painkillers is an indirect evaluation of postoperative pain severity. Several reports conclude PRA reduces the need for painkillers after surgery. According to Martin Walz, consumption of analgesics in the postoperative period of 143 procedures in 130 patients was only 6 mg of piritramide. This represents a low need for medication [10]. Carlos Serra also reported a low need for painkillers in the postoperative days [11]. In a visual analog scale (VAS—1–10) PRA patients report a mean of 3.4 ± 1 at postoperative day 1. In TLAdr, the VAS pain score rises to 4.2 ± 1 ($p < 0.05$) [24]. Using the same scale, Kiriakopoulos concluded that PRA caused less pain than TLAdr in postoperative days 1 and 3 ($p < 0.001$) [17]. According to Cabalag, 26 patients out of 49 (52%) needed no postoperative analgesic medication following PRA [12]. All these data support the very low postoperative pain associated with PRA.

In prospective and retrospective studies, PRA is associated with less postoperative pain than TLAdr [12, 13, 17, 24–26]. A comparative study between the two techniques concluded that 37.5% of patients submitted to TLAdr requested postoperative opioids, contrasting to 3% of patients treated by PRA ($p < 0.001$) [19]. Additionally, shoulder-tip pain is a rarity after PRA ($p < 0.001$) [19, 24]. In 2021, a systematic review and meta-analysis which included 800 patients confirmed less postoperative pain after PRA comparing to TLAdr ($p = 0.026$) [26].

11.6 In-Hospital Days and Recovery to Normal Activity

Following the first 143 procedures during a five-year period, Walz reported a median hospitalization of 3 days [10]. A mean of 3 days for in-hospital length of stay was also reported by Nancy Perrier's group in the USA [16]. In 2015, Kiriakopoulos reported a length of stay of 2.1 days in a group of 17 patients [17]. A mean postoperative in-hospital length of stay of 2.2 days was reported by CE Costa Almeida in 2018 [5]. Two years later, CE Costa Almeida reduced the in-hospital postoperative length of stay to a mean of 1.7 days. This reduction was due to a shorter postoperative period for pheochromocytoma patients after learning that PRA was not causing hemodynamic instability. The initial four postoperative in-hospital days were reduced to only 2 days (one in the ICU and one in the surgery ward) [15]. A median length of stay of 1 day was reported in Cabalag's study. In this work, 8 of the 49 patients were discharged on the same day [12] (Table 11.1). According to this data, PRA can eventually be performed as ambulatory surgery on suitable patients.

PRA is associated with a shorter time to first oral intake (4.4 h) and a shorter time to ambulation (6.1 h) as compared to TLAdr [19]. PRA also promotes faster recovery to normal activity than TLAdr [3, 5, 12, 25, 27]. These are major advantages as they can reduce the days of absence from work.

11.7 Learning Curve

PRA has a short learning curve [12, 14, 15]. A shorter learning curve is possible if the surgeon is already skilled and experienced in other laparoscopic surgeries [13]. This is the advantage of performing different procedures—skills acquired in one are useful in another. Operative time and complication rate are usually the two factors studied when analyzing the learning curve of any procedure [13]. Several reports have concluded that, with experience, there is a decrease in operative time. In a 2006 analysis of 560 PRA, Walz observed a gradual decrease in operative time from 106 ± 46 min to 40 ± 15 min. Additionally, there was the need to use a fourth trocar in 29/560 procedures, but only once in the last 250 PRA [4]. In 2018, Alesina et al. reduced the mean operative time to 45 min after 2310 procedures, with a complication rate below 1% [3]. In a study by van Uitert, operative time consistently decreased after each of the first 3 groups of 20 patients. Operative time reached a median of 60 min after 40 procedures and was found to plateau after 70 cases [21]. Similar results were reported by Barczynski [28]. Comparing the first group with the second group of 50 procedures, there was a decrease in mean operative time ($p < 0.001$). After 60 cases, operative time stabilized at 65 min. Although conversion and blood loss were lower in the second group, there was no statistical significance [28]. In a consensus paper by the European Society of Endocrine Surgeons (ESES), the learning curve for PRA is estimated to be 20–40 cases [29]. However, according to Cabalag's results, it is possible to lower the learning curve below 20 procedures [12]. Operative time decreased by 4.2 min/case in the first 10 cases and decreased by 2.3 min/case in the next 5 cases. After performing 15 PRA, operative time stabilized in 61 min, with the same rate of complications and the same outcomes [12]. Bakkar et al. lowered the learning curve even more. They reported a mean operative time of less than 1 h only after 14 cases [23].

The learning curve is difficult to assess. What is the endpoint of the learning curve? Possibly, it is that of reaching a plateau in operative time with a low rate of complications and good outcomes. Many factors influence the length of that curve, namely: the surgeon, training opportunities, tumor pathology, patient characteristics, available equipment, hospital, and case volume [13]. The number of procedures necessary for a surgeon to acquire competence in PRA is a matter of debate. It cannot be a fixed number, since different surgeons have different skills, and each one of them has his or her own learning pace. In four different centers, surgeons reached competence in PRA after 24, 29, 40, and 42 procedures [3]. If a surgeon has experience in laparoscopic surgery (colorectal, hepatobiliary, hernia, etc.) the learning curve will be shorter. This idea was confirmed in 2020, in a publication by CE Costa Almeida [15]. After performing 20 cases, his group matched the outcomes (morbidity and mortality) of more experienced surgeons, with a lower mean operative time of 38.9 min. The expertise gained from different laparoscopic surgeries lowered the learning curve to less than 20

procedures [15]. Surgeons with laparoscopic skills will be able to easily learn and perform PRA [20].

Patient selection is especially important at the beginning of the learning curve. Obesity is not absolutely prohibited but operating on patients with BMI ≥35 can be very challenging. Obese patients should be avoided when starting the learning curve. If possible, patients suffering from Cushing's Syndrome should also not be the first cases due to the amount of fatty tissue with which the surgeon will have to deal [14, 24].

Equipment and hospital are both factors that should be easily overcome. An adequate operation table for correct patient positioning is crucial. Trocars, instruments, energy devices, and cameras all work together to help the surgeon perform a fast, safe, and efficient PRA. Hospital Administration Boards should rely on surgeons to decide which instruments and laparoscopic cameras to buy. Unfortunately, this is not always the rule. The lack of knowledge of the administrations and the constant aim to save money can preclude the practice of safe and efficient medicine. Only with good and adequate equipment can a patient be offered the best treatment solution. This is the only way to achieve the best outcomes, decrease complications, decrease in-hospital days, and avoid rehospitalizations. High-quality medicine will always be the cheapest medicine.

A minimum annual workload related to improved final outcomes is still a matter of debate. ESES consensus paper from 2019 presents a minimum of 6 procedures/year, increasing to 12 adrenalectomies/year for adrenocortical cancer [29]. In this definition, surgeons' experience and laparoscopic skills must be considered since they have a positive impact on the final outcomes and learning curve. Establishing a minimum number of procedures is something difficult, probably unfair, and utopic. In some cases, the centralization of procedures will limit the accessibility to the best treatment for patients living in remote areas. An honest outcome evaluation must be the key point to establishing who should keep operating adrenal, and who should receive updated training and re-tutorized by an experienced surgeon.

It must be highlighted that learning the technique from an experienced surgeon is crucial for these results [29]. Meeting and working with an expert for a specific period is of paramount importance. Watching and assisting an expert performing several PRAs is the best way to learn the tips and tricks of the technique. Although not mandatory, to have an experienced surgeon by your side during the first procedures might be of good value. Authors reporting operative times <60 min after 14, 15, 20, and 40 cases learned how to perform PRA from an expert [13]. Additionally, if the surgeon has the laparoscopic surgical skills learned from other procedures, it will not take long for him or her to achieve the outcomes of more experienced surgeons.

11.8   Final Notes

PRA is a safe and feasible technique, with several advantages over anterior and lateral laparoscopic approaches. PRA gives direct access to the adrenal gland while avoiding intra-abdominal incursion and the need for organ mobilization. It is an ideal technique for patients with previous abdominal surgeries and reduces the risk of viscera injuries. It is a good technique for lesions up to 6–8 cm because larger tumors have an increased risk of cancer, and they are difficult to manipulate without capsule rupture [4, 20]. Complications can occur in <1–16%, but most of them are minor and temporary. Additionally, the overall complication rate decreases with experience [3–5, 16, 22]. Very obese patients (BMI > 45) are not good candidates for this technique, considering that, even with high pressures of CO_2 it is not possible to have a good working space [4, 16, 20]. Operative time for PRA is identical to laparoscopic cholecystectomy and endoscopic hernia repair. The author has a mean operative time of 38.9 min after 20 cases [15]. Although the learning curve is still a matter of debate, PRA is an easy-to-learn technique if the surgeon already has experience in laparoscopic surgery [5]. Patients submitted to PRA report an excellent satisfaction with the outcomes (symptoms and cosmesis) [18]. These results prove the feasibility, safety, and effectiveness of PRA.

Systematic reviews and randomized trials support PRA over TLAdr [19, 24, 26, 27]. The former is associated with a significantly shorter operative time, lower blood loss, less postoperative pain, shorter time to first oral intake, shorter in-hospital length of stay, and better cost-benefit ($p < 0.001$). Morbidity and conversion rate are similar in both techniques, but PRA has fewer incisional hernias (0% vs 16.1%). In conclusion, PRA should become the new gold standard for adrenal surgery [13].

References

1. Higashihara E, Tanaka Y, Horie S, Aruga S, Nutahara K, Homma Y, et al. A case report of laparoscopic adrenalectomy. Nihon Hinyokika Gakkai Zasshi. 1992;83(7):1130–3.
2. Gagner M, Lacroix A, Bolté E. Laparoscopic adrenalectomy in Cushing's syndrome and pheochromocytoma. N Engl J Med. 1992;327(14):1033.
3. Alesina PF. Retroperitoneal adrenalectomy-learning curve, practical tips and tricks, what limits its wider uptake. Gland Surg. 2019;8(Suppl 1):S36–40.
4. Walz MK, Alesina PF, Wenger FA, Deligiannis A, Szuczik E, Petersenn S, et al. Posterior retroperitoneoscopic adrenalectomy-results of 560 procedures in 520 patients. Surgery. 2006;140(6):943–8.
5. Costa Almeida CE, Caroço T, Silva MA, Albano MN, Louro JM, Carvalho LF, et al. Posterior retroperitoneoscopic adrenalectomy—Case series. Int J Surg Case Rep. 2018;51:174–7.
6. Lee CR, Walz MK, Park S, Park JH, Jeong JS, Lee SH, et al. A comparative study of the transperitoneal and posterior retroperitoneal approaches for laparoscopic adrenalectomy for adrenal tumors. Ann Surg Oncol. 2012;19(8):2629–34.
7. Uchida M, Imaide Y, Yoneda K, Uehara H, Ukimura O, Itoh Y, et al. Endoscopic adrenalectomy by retroperitoneal approach for primary aldosteronism. Hinyokika Kiyo. 1994;40(1):43–6.
8. Johansson K, Anderberg B, Asberg B, Endoscopic retroperitoneal adrenalectomy. A technique useful for surgery of minor tumors. Lakartidningen. 1994;91(37):3278–81.
9. Whittle DE, Schroeder D, Purchas SH, Sivakumaran P, Conaglen JV. Laparoscopic retroperitoneal left adrenalectomy in a patient with Cushing's syndrome. Aust N Z J Surg. 1994;64(5):375–6.
10. Walz MK, Peitgen K, Walz MV, Hoermann R, Saller B, Giebler RM, et al. Posterior retroperitoneoscopic

adrenalectomy: lessons learned within five years. World J Surg. 2001;25(6):728–34.

11. Serra C, Pereira Canudo A, Silvestre dos Santos A. Adrenalectomia posterior retroperitoneoscópica – introdução da técnica num hospital generalista. Revista Portuguesa de Endocrinologia, Diabetes e Metabolismo. 2016;11(2):253–7.

12. Cabalag MS, Mann GB, Gorelik A, Miller JA. Posterior retroperitoneoscopic adrenalectomy: outcomes and lessons learned from initial 50 cases. ANZ J Surg. 2015;85(6):478–82.

13. Li R, Miller JA. Evaluating the learning curve for posterior retroperitoneoscopic adrenalectomy. Ann Laparosc Endosc Surg. 2017;2:169.

14. Gimm O, Duh QY. Challenges of training in adrenal surgery. Gland Surg. 2019;8(Suppl 1):S3–9.

15. Costa Almeida CE, Caroço T, Silva MA, Baião JM, Costa A, Albano MN, et al. An update of posterior retroperitoneoscopic adrenalectomy—case series. Int J Surg Case Rep. 2020;71:120–5.

16. Perrier ND, Kennamer DL, Bao R, Jimenez C, Grubbs EG, Lee JE, et al. Posterior retroperitoneoscopic adrenalectomy: preferred technique for removal of benign tumors and isolated metastases. Ann Surg. 2008;248(4):666–74.

17. Kiriakopoulos A, Petralias A, Linos D. Posterior retroperitoneoscopic versus laparoscopic adrenalectomy in sporadic and MENIIA pheochromocytomas. Surg Endosc. 2015;29(8):2164–70.

18. Porpiglia F, Fiori C, Bertolo R, Cattaneo G, Amparore D, Morra I, et al. Mini-retroperitoneoscopic adrenal ectomy: our experience after 50 procedures. Urology. 2014;84(3):596–601.

19. Barczyński M, Konturek A, Nowak W. Randomized clinical trial of posterior retroperitoneoscopic adrenalectomy versus lateral transperitoneal laparoscopic adrenalectomy with a 5-year follow-up. Ann Surg. 2014;260(5):740–7.

20. Dickson PV, Jimenez C, Chisholm GB, Kennamer DL, Ng C, Grubbs EG, et al. Posterior retroperitoneoscopic adrenalectomy: a contemporary American experience. J Am Coll Surg. 2011;212(4):659–65.

21. van Uitert A, d'Ancona FCH, Deinum J, Timmers HJLM, Langenhuijsen JF. Evaluating the learning curve for retroperitoneoscopic adrenalectomy in a high-volume center for laparoscopic adrenal surgery. Surg Endosc. 2017;31(7):2771–5.

22. Kumar M, Kumar R, Hemal AK, Gupta NP. Complications of retroperitoneoscopic surgery at one centre. BJU Int. 2001;87(7):607–12.

23. Bakkar S, Materazzi G, Fregoli L, Papini P, Miccoli P. Posterior retroperitonoscopic adrenalectomy; a back door access with an unusually rapid learning curve. Updat Surg. 2017;69(2):235–9.

24. Kozłowski T, Choromanska B, Wojskowicz P, Astapczyk K, Łukaszewicz J, Rutkowski D, et al. Laparoscopic adrenalectomy: lateral transperitoneal versus posterior retroperitoneal approach—prospective randomized trial. Wideochir Inne Tech Maloinwazyjne. 2019;14(2):160–9.

25. Walz MK. Minimally invasive adrenal gland surgery: transperitoneal or retroperitoneal approach? Chirurg. 2012;83(6):536–45.

26. Meng C, Du C, Peng L, Li J, Li J, Li Y, et al. Comparison of posterior retroperitoneoscopic adrenalectomy versus lateral transperitoneal laparoscopic adrenalectomy for adrenal Tumors: a systematic review and meta-analysis. Front Oncol. 2021;11:667985.

27. Chai YJ, Kwon H, Yu HW, Kim SJ, Choi JY, Lee KE, et al. Systematic review of surgical approaches for adrenal tumors: lateral transperitoneal versus posterior retroperitoneal and laparoscopic versus robotic adrenalectomy. Int J Endocrinol. 2014;2014:918346.

28. Barczyński M, Konturek A, Gołkowski F, Cichoń S, Huszno B, Peitgen K, et al. Posterior retroperitoneoscopic adrenalectomy: a comparison between the initial experience in the invention phase and introductory phase of the new surgical technique. World J Surg. 2007;31(1):65–71.

29. Mihai R, Donatini G, Vidal O, Brunaud L. Volume-outcome correlation in adrenal surgery—an ESES consensus statement. Langenbeck's Arch Surg. 2019;404(7):795–806.

Robotic Surgery and Innovation

12

Murat Özdemir, Varlık Erol, and Özer Makay

12.1 Introduction

The emergence of robot-assisted surgery has brought some advantages to minimally invasive surgery. Compared to classical laparoscopic systems, robotic systems allow for three-dimensional visualization with more pleasing contrast and color resolution. In addition, they are equipped with sensitive instruments with high mobility that can work in smaller areas. However, this better technology comes at a higher overall cost. Another disadvantage is the need for a well-trained surgeon and supporting team to use the system, which can be complex. The first use of robotic technology in adrenal gland surgery was made in 1999 by Piazza et al. in Italy [1]. As the robotic system became widespread globally, publications with larger numbers of cases followed. In the current literature, transabdominal lateral robotic adrenalectomy (TL-RA) seems to be a more commonly used technique than robotic posterior retroperitoneal adrenalectomy (RPRA). A recently published EUROCRINE study com-pared robot-assisted and conventional laparoscopic adrenalectomy [2]. EUROCRINE is an online endocrine surgical quality registry that aims to decrease mortality in the surgical care of patients with endocrine tumors, with a special focus on rare tumors, by means of an international database based in Europe. In the aforementioned study, data from 46 centers registered in the system were examined. The authors excluded retroperitoneal cases because the number of RPRAs was only six. Vatansever et al. studied 1005 patients, 816 of whom were laparoscopic and 189 were robot-assisted adrenalectomy. The authors suggested that robotic adrenalectomy could be considered a preferred approach in more challenging and difficult cases, including large (>50 mm) and functioning (e.g., pheochromocytoma) tumors and obese patients. In conclusion, analysis of the EUROCRINE database supports that, beyond being safe and effective, robot-assisted adrenalectomies show lower complication rates and shorter postoperative durations of stay [2]. Although it is not very common in the EUROCRINE information system, RPRA has been performed in many centers in increasing numbers since 2010, when it was first described in the literature. In this section, the surgical technique of RPRA and the results of this technique will be discussed.

M. Özdemir · Ö. Makay (✉)
Department of General Surgery, Division of Endocrine Surgery, Ege University Hospital, Izmir, Turkey

V. Erol
Department of General Surgery, Medicana International Hospital, Izmir, Turkey

© The Author(s), under exclusive license to Springer Nature Switzerland AG 2023
C. E. Costa Almeida (ed.), *Posterior Retroperitoneoscopic Adrenalectomy*,
https://doi.org/10.1007/978-3-031-19995-0_12

12.2 Surgical Technique of Robotic Posterior Retroperitoneal Adrenalectomy

Many minimally invasive techniques are used for the surgical treatment of adrenal gland diseases. One of these techniques is RPRA, which many centers successfully apply, and is a safe, feasible, and effective method [3]. This approach ensures avoidance of the peritoneal cavity, which is the main advantage. Not entering the peritoneal cavity reduces complications associated with intraperitoneal access, such as visceral injury, intraperitoneal bleeding, and adhesion formation. Therefore, RPRA may be the preferred approach, especially in patients who require intervention on bilateral adrenal glands and in patients who have had more than one abdominal surgery—in these cases, intraperitoneal surgery may be more difficult due to previous adhesion formation. However, the most significant shortcoming of RPRA is the limitation in the working area, which increases the technical difficulties of the operation.

12.3 Preoperative Preparation and Setup of the Patient

The RPRA technique is slightly modified compared to the conventional approach. Robotic surgery can be performed with one of the DaVinci robotic surgery systems (Intuitive Surgical Sarl, Aubonne, Switzerland). The system consists of a 4-arm robotic manipulator and remote control surgical console. Surgery is performed under general anesthesia. Preoperative preparation and patient positioning are the same as posterior retroperitoneoscopic adrenalectomy (PRA). The robotic approach provides enough working space and facilitates orientation by providing readily identifiable anatomical landmarks and better visualization of surrounding anatomical structures.

The patient is carefully placed in a prone jack-knife position (Fig. 12.1). Attention should be paid to pressure points, and necessary places (especially the axilla) should be supported appropriately with pillows and gels. The retroperitoneal space is entered through a 1.5–2 cm transverse incision, placed just beneath the lowest tip of the 12th rib. Then, the trocar is replaced with a dissecting balloon under direct view to generate an adequate working space. After that, a medial 12-mm-long trocar is placed along the lateral border of the paraspinous muscles. Next, two 8-mm robotic trocars are applied, one lateral to the 12th rib port site and one medial approximately 3 cm below the junction of the 12th rib and the spine. A 5-mm inferior port is often placed 3–5 cm (as far away as possible from each other, attempting to prevent instrument collision) caudad to the central port site and used for the assistant port (retractor, suction, or irrigator device). The role of the assistant at the surgical table is to change the robotic instruments when necessary, assist in dissection from the assistant's port, attach the clip to the adrenal vein, seal with the vessel

Fig. 12.1 Patient positioning for RPRA

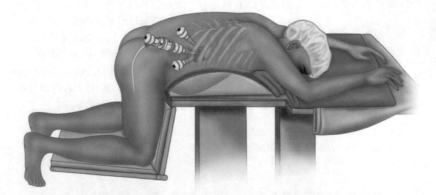

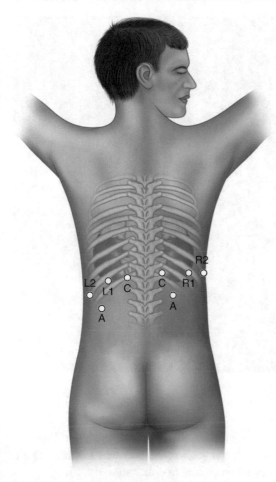

Fig. 12.2 Port placement for RPRA. A—assistant port, C—camera, L1, L2—robotic trocars (left side), R1, R2—robotic trocars (right side)

the port application, a 30-degree robotic endoscope is inserted, and the cavity is carefully inspected to exclude any iatrogenic injuries or to check for other retroperitoneal masses. At this point, the robotic unit is docked, and the primary surgeon moves to the operating console (Fig. 12.3).

Once the robotic unit is docked, the 8-mm robotic cadiere forceps are used on the left-sided port and the 8-mm robotic cautery hook is used on the right-side port. This may change according to the surgeon's preference. The 30-degree camera is looking down from this point, and dissection is carried out from lateral to medial, detaching the tissue above the kidney. Next, the assistant retracts the kidney caudally. The surgeon subsequently dissects the adrenal gland and the tissue surrounding it from the superior aspect of the kidney. First, the right or left adrenal vein is identified medially, extending from the adrenal gland to the vena cava or renal vein, respectively. Then, the adrenal vein is carefully dissected and clipped (using the robotic clip applier or standard laparoscopic clips) or ligated with a vessel sealer—placed by the bedside assistant through the 5-mm assistant port. The adrenal gland is then removed from its retroperitoneal attachments. For hemostasis control, before the mass is removed from the retroperitoneal area, it is advised to wait 3–4 minutes after the retroperitoneal gas is evacuated and recheck the operation site. After the adrenalectomy is complete, the robotic unit is undocked. The gland is removed using a specimen retrieval bag and delivered via the 12-mm middle port by extending the port site incision at the skin and fascia, as necessary. After the operative site is irrigated and suctioned, the trocars are removed. The trocar sites are closed appropriately. The patient is then placed supine, extubated, and taken to the recovery room in a stable condition.

sealing device, and perform the wash-aspiration process (Fig. 12.2). Pneumoretroperitoneum is established with CO_2 insufflation, maintained at 15–20 mmHg throughout the procedure. A 30-degree non-robotic endoscope is introduced looking up. Gerota's retroperitoneal fascia is then taken down without injuring surrounding structures or violating the peritoneal layer laterally using a blunt laparoscopic grasper. After

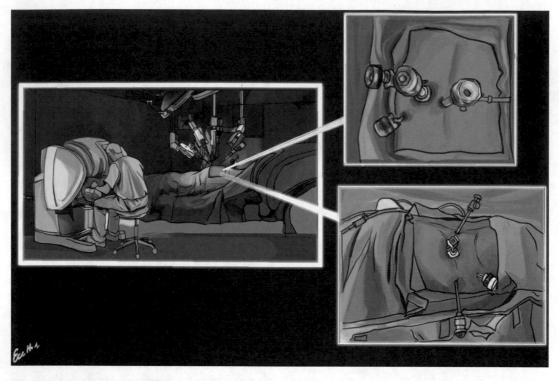

Fig. 12.3 Ports in place for RPRA

12.4 Evidence Regarding Robotic Posterior Retroperitoneal Adrenalectomy

12.4.1 Case Series

The surgical technique of RPRA was first described by Berber et al. in 2010 in a series of 8 patients [4]. The mean operative time in these first series was 214.8 min, docking time was 21.7 min, and console time was 97.1 min. In the first few cases, the docking time lasted 60 minutes, but later on, this time could be reduced to 7 min. The mean blood loss was 24 ml, and the patients were discharged from the hospital within 24 h. The highlight in this first series was the length of the operation time, which was quite long compared to the conventional retroperitoneoscopic adrenalectomy data.

Also in 2010, a 6-patient study (one of the first RPRA series) was published by Ludwing et al. [5]. In this study, the mean operation time was 121 min, the console time was 57 minutes, the docking time was 14 minutes, the blood loss was <60 ml, and the hospital stay was 1.3 days. There was no morbidity in either study [4, 5].

After these initial reports, Dickson et al. published a series of 30 RPRA procedures performed on 28 consecutive patients (26 unilateral and 2 bilateral) [6]. Indications for adrenalectomy included pheochromocytoma, hyperaldosteronism, hypercortisolism, oligometastases, and nonfunctional tumors. The mean tumor size in the study was 3.8 ± 1.6 cm, and the mean body mass index was 30.7 ± 6.5 kg/m^2. The mean operative time for unilateral total adrenalectomy was 154 ± 43 minutes, the estimated blood loss (EBL) was 28.3 ± 50.9 ml, and the conversion rate to the open procedure was zero. Three patients had perioperative complications. These complications were reported as pneumothorax, urinary retention, and retroperitoneal hematoma requiring postoperative blood transfusion. In addition, cortex-sparing RPRA was performed for pheochromocytoma in four patients with MEN2A in this series. One of these patients underwent right adrenalectomy and left cortex-sparing adrenalectomy. No recurrent pheochromocytoma was observed in any patient during follow-up longer than 6 months. In addition, average serum cortisol values were found in the patient who underwent the bilateral procedure. Based on their early experience, the authors commented that robotic surgery might better preserve the vascularized residue during minimally invasive cortical sparing adrenalectomy thanks to its three-dimensional visualization capabilities, ergonomic design, enhanced visualization tools compared to those in standard endoscopic operations, and a more flexible approach to dissection. In addition, the fluorescence imaging ability of the robotic system may help visualize the integrity of the blood supply of the remnant adrenal tissue in such cases [7].

12.4.2 Laparoscopic Versus Robotic Posterior Retroperitoneal Adrenalectomy

In their 2012 study, Ağcaoğlu et al. compared 31 laparoscopic posterior retroperitoneal adrenalectomy (LPRA) and 31 RPRA cases [8]. Tumor size, blood loss, hospital stay, and skin-to-skin surgery times were similar between the two groups. However, after an initial learning curve of 10 cases, operative times were significantly shorter in the robotic group (139 vs. 167 min, $p = 0.046$), including robotic insertion times ranging from 5 to 30 min. In addition, pain scores on the postoperative first day were lower in the robotic group than in the laparoscopic retroperitoneal group ($p = 0.008$). The authors attributed this to the shorter operative time and less pressure on the incisions due to their articulating instruments.

In 2019, in a study published by Kim et al., LPRA was performed on 169 patients and RPRA on 61 patients [9]. There was no difference between the two groups regarding tumor size, BMI, EBL, or hospital stay. However, a significant difference between the two groups was found in the mean operation time (117 minutes for the LPRA group vs. 142 min for the RPRA group, $p = 0.006$). Furthermore, in the LPRA group, there was a positive correlation between operative time and male gender, tumor size, and pheochromocytoma. In RPRA, tumor size and pheochromocytoma affected the operation time. When the adrenal tumor size was ≤5.5 cm, a shorter operative time was registered in LPRA than RPRA ($p = 0.001$). There was no significant difference between LPRA and RPRA operation times when the tumor size was >5.5 cm ($p = 0.102$).

In a 51-patient study published by Fu et al. in 2020 comparing LPRA ($n = 32$) and RPRA ($n = 19$) only in patients with pheochromocytoma, the incidence of hemodynamic instability was lower in the RPRA group (26.3% vs. 56.2%, $p = 0.038$) [10]. In addition, in the RPRA group, the EBL (100 ml vs. 200 ml, $p = 0.042$) and hospital stay (5 days vs. 6 days, $p = 0.02$) were significantly lower than in the LPRA group.

In a study published by Ma et al. in 2021 comparing 86 RPRA and 315 LPRA patients, no difference was found regarding demographic and tumor characteristics between the two groups [11]. However, the mean postoperative stay (3 vs. 4 days, $p = 0.001$) was significantly shorter in the RPRA group. In addition, there was no difference between the two groups regarding the median operative time (100 vs. 110 min, $p = 0.554$), the median EBL (50 ml vs. 50 ml, $p = 0.730$), transfusion rate ($p = 0.497$), and incidence of postoperative complications ($p = 0.428$).

In 2013, Park et al. carried out "single-port" RPRA on five patients with adrenal cortical adenoma. The series had a mean operative time of 159.4 ± 57.6 (103–245) minutes and a mean EBL of 46.0 ± 56.8 (5–120) ml. Neither conversion to open surgery nor postoperative complications were reported in any patient [12].

12.4.3 Robotic Posterior Retroperitoneal Adrenalectomy Versus Transabdominal Lateral Robotic Adrenalectomy

In 2017, Kahramangil et al. compared RPRA and TL-RA cases [13]. As a result, there were 188 robotic adrenalectomy patients, 12 of whom underwent bilateral surgeries. In addition, 110 patients were operated on using the transabdominal lateral approach and 78 using the posterior retroperitoneal approach. When both groups were compared, in patients of similar age and gender, the tumor size was larger (4.2 ± 2.5 vs. 3.3 ± 2.0 cm, $p = 0.01$) and BMI was higher (29.2 ± 4.7 vs. 32.3 ± 8.1) in the TL-RA group. Furthermore, the operation time was significantly shorter in the RPRA group (136.3 ± 38.7 vs. 154.6 ± 48.4 min, $p = 0.005$). The authors stated that this difference was due to the shorter exposure time (32.8 ± 17.3 vs. 43.3 ± 14.9 minutes, $p = 0.001$). There was no difference in the EBL, conversion to open surgery, and length of hospital stay between the two approaches. Complications were observed in nine patients (the most common was urinary tract infection), similar in both groups. The authors reported no mortality. The pain score was higher in the TL-RA group on the postoperative first day ($p = 0.001$) and similar between the two groups on day 14. As a result of the study, the authors emphasized that the postoperative outcomes of both approaches were excellent and recommended that suitable patients should undergo RPRA in experienced centers because of the shorter operation time and lower postoperative pain.

12.4.4 Cost Analysis

Cost has been shown to be one of the most critical disadvantages of robotic surgery in general. However, studies have demonstrated that the multidisciplinary use of a robotic system and the increase in the number of surgeries performed to reduce costs. In a cost analysis report by Barbash et al., the additional cost of using a robot for unilateral adrenalectomies was estimated to range between 1400 and 2900 USD, or about 10–20% of the cost of the entire procedure [14].

Ma et al. also performed a detailed cost analysis of LPRA and RPRA. While the total cost of hospitalization was 8122 USD in the RPRA group, this cost was reported as 4108 USD in the LPRA group ($p = 0.001$) [11]. On the other hand, despite the fact that Ağcaoğlu et al. did not perform a detailed cost analysis in their study, the authors stated that the cost was approximately 900–950 USD per robotic procedure. They also argued that anesthesia costs for various general surgical procedures are 16–21 USD per minute and that RPRA can reduce the cost by shortening the operation time [8].

Acknowledgments The authors thank Bilge Çandereli, Ece Horasanlı, and Ceren Taşan for their wonderful drawing.

Conflict of Interest The authors have no conflicts of interest to declare.

References

1. Piazza L, Caragliano P, Scardilli M, Sgroi AV, Marino G, Giannone G. Laparoscopic robot-assisted right adrenalectomy and left ovariectomy (case reports). Chir Ital. 1999;51(6):465–6.
2. Vatansever S, Nordenström E, Raffaelli M, Brunaud L, Makay Ö, EUROCRINE Council. Robot-assisted versus conventional laparoscopic adrenalectomy: results from the EUROCRINE surgical registry. Surgery. 2022;171(5):1224–30.
3. Makay O, Erol V, Ozdemir M. Robotic adrenalectomy. Gland Surg. 2019;8(Suppl 1):S10–6.
4. Berber E, Mitchell J, MilasM SA. Robotic posterior retroperitoneal adrenalectomy: operative technique. Arch Surg. 2010;145(8):781–4.
5. Ludwig AT, Wagner KR, Lowry PS, Papaconstantinou HT, Lairmore TC. Robot-assisted posterior retroperitoneoscopic adrenalectomy. J Endourol. 2010;24(8):1307–14.
6. Dickson PV, Alex GC, Grubbs EG, Jimenez C, Lee JE, Perrier ND. Robotic-assisted retroperitoneoscopic adrenalectomy: making a good procedure even better. Am Surg. 2013;79(1):84–9.
7. Agcaoglu O, Kulle CB, Berber E. Indocyanine green fluorescence imaging for robotic adrenalectomy. Gland Surg. 2020;9(3):849–52.

8. Agcaoglu O, Aliyev S, Karabulut K, Siperstein A, Berber E. Robotic vs. laparoscopic posterior retroperitoneal adrenalectomy. Arch Surg. 2012;147(3):272–5.

9. Kim WW, Lee YM, Chung KW, Hong SJ, Sung TY. Comparison of robotic posterior retroperitoneal adrenalectomy over laparoscopic posterior retroperitoneal adrenalectomy: a single tertiary Center experience. Int J Endocrinol. 2019;2019:9012910.

10. Fu SQ, Zhuang CS, Yang XR, Xie WJ, Gong BB, Liu YF, et al. Comparison of robot-assisted retroperitoneal laparoscopic adrenalectomy versus retroperitoneal laparoscopic adrenalectomy for large pheochromocytoma: a single-centre retrospective study. BMC Surg. 2020;20(1):227.

11. Ma W, Mao Y, Dai J, Alimu P, Zhuo R, He W, et al. Propensity score matched analysis comparing robotic-assisted with laparoscopic posterior retroperitoneal adrenalectomy. J Investig Surg. 2021;34(11):1248–53.

12. Park JH, Kim SY, Lee CR, Park S, Jeong JS, Kang SW, et al. Robot-assisted posterior retroperitoneoscopic adrenalectomy using single-port access: technical feasibility and preliminary results. Ann Surg Oncol. 2013;20(8):2741–5.

13. Kahramangil B, Berber E. Comparison of posterior retroperitoneal and transabdominal lateral approaches in robotic adrenalectomy: an analysis of 200 cases. Surg Endosc. 2018;32(4):1984–9.

14. Barbash GI, Glied SA. New technology and health care costs—the case of robot-assisted surgery. N Engl J Med. 2010;363(8):701–4.

Printed in the United States
by Baker & Taylor Publisher Services